LIVING
IN THE
LIGHTNING

Wild Lace (poems)

My Father Spoke of His Riches (poems)

The Peas Belong on the Eye Level (poems)

Eclipse (poems)

Savage Grace (coauthored with Steven M. L.

Aronson/nonfiction)

Alien Ink: The FBI's War on Freedom of Expression

(nonfiction)

The Girl Who Died Twice: The Libby Zion Case and

the Hidden Hazards of Hospitals (nonfiction)

LIVING
IN THE
LIGHTNING

A CANCER JOURNAL

Natalie Robins

RUTGERS UNIVERSITY PRESS

NEW BRUNSWICK, NEW JERSEY, AND LONDON

Library of Congress Cataloging-in-Publication Data

Robins, Natalie S.
    Living in the lightning : a cancer journal / Natalie Robins.
        p.   cm.
    Includes bibliographical references.
    ISBN 0-8135-2664-7 (cloth : alk. paper). — ISBN 0-8135-2665-5
(pbk. : alk. paper)
    1. Robins, Natalie. S.—Health.   2. Lymphomas—Patients—New York
(State)—New York—Biography.   I. Title.
RC280.L9R62 1999
362.1'9699446'0092—dc21
    [b]   98-37622
                                                                      CIP

British Cataloging-in-Publication data for this book is available from the British
Library

Manufactured in the United States of America

In Memory of Karen Avenoso,

1967–1998

A young journalist I knew
only through her gifted, brave,
and far-too-brief career,
which ended because of cancer

CONTENTS

LIVING
IN THE
LIGHTNING

INTRODUCTION

I have always written to save myself—from sadness, loss, despair, pain, or even ignorance. I believe that writers choose the subjects they do to teach themselves something about the world around them, or within them, and in doing so, they also teach things to the world. It's a simple, elegant exchange.

After the death of my newborn daughter in 1976, I wrote a long series of poems I called *Birth Elegy*, which I included in my final book of poems, *Eclipse*, published in 1981. I say my final book of poems because I have since become a nonfiction writer, and write now more to educate myself. Or so I like to think.

My most recent book, *The Girl Who Died Twice: The Libby Zion Case and the Hidden Hazards of Hospitals*, about a landmark malpractice case and the state of medical education in our country today, was published in 1995, two months before my cancer diagnosis. Indeed, I would later find out that I had been living with my cancer without knowing it for the previous three to five years, a not uncommon situation I would also discover, especially with indolent forms of non-Hodgkin's lymphoma, a cancer of the body's lymph system.

For two years, I had felt what at first was a ridge or unevenness, then a small bump (for some reason I never referred to it as a lump) in my lower back. I became obsessed with it, although I didn't go to a doctor. I looked at it in the mirror all the time, turning this way and that way to see if it was really "something" or not. In time, I showed it to my husband and some friends, including a few doctors. Everyone tried to reassure me. No one was worried, except me. But over the summer of 1995, it seemed to be growing, and to be darkening. I described it to myself as "getting bolder." Yet I still thought: could I be imagining this? Was I just having prepublication anxieties because my book was about to be published? Then, when I was bending over while trying on a pair of jeans in a store, I felt a piercing, tear-jerking pain in my lower back. I thought it must be from the needlelike point of one of those security devices attached to clothes, or from some misplaced straight pin. But it wasn't. I checked carefully. Frightened, I finally decided to call my internist. He thought the bump was probably nothing, but said that if I was concerned about it (and I was) I should see a plastic surgeon to have it removed. Finally, in October, I made an appointment with one.

The plastic surgeon did not like what he saw, and immediately took two biopsies. He had a lot of trouble with the first one, a fine-needle biopsy, because the specimen was "too thick," and had "too many cells." He later performed a more successful tissue biopsy. He rushed the results to me (and my internist), and became the person who gave me the first indication that my bump was far from nothing.

It was, in fact, cancer.

Some of my friends are doctors, and some of my doctors are friends. I live near several large New York City medical centers, and because of this, many doctors live where I live—in the Riverdale section of the Bronx, a tree-filled, villagelike community close to the Hudson River. My comfort around doctors helped when I researched my book about the Zion case, and by the time I finished writing it, I felt pretty familiar with the world of medicine.

While I was annoyed at the doctors who had not taken my bump seriously, I was never deeply angry at them. I talked to them about everything I was feeling, and was honest (but not hurtful). After all, who wants to think that a bump—or lump, I can call it that now—especially one in an unusual place like the lower back, is cancerous? I was programmed to look for suspicious lumps only in my breasts or armpits, not my back. (But I certainly don't think like this anymore, and neither do my doctors.)

I consider myself lucky, because even if my cancer had been discovered much earlier, my treatment probably would not have begun until it actually did anyway. Most other cancers do not have this "watch and wait" option. Still, I realize once again, and more than ever, that no one cares about my body as much as I do. I know my body best, and must continue to trust my instincts about everything right and wrong with it.

Doctors have far more medical knowledge than I do, yet I know the map (me) better than they ever can. But together we will find our way. This is what is most critical in any medical circumstance— the flu, a bee sting, diabetes, surgery, or yes, cancer—that doctor-patient togetherness grows and grows, like a summer garden. It needs occasional weeding and pruning, but with steady, conscientious care it can thrive (like a cancer patient).

At first I resisted even keeping a journal because I couldn't reconcile the informal, spontaneous aspect of a journal with my belief that real writing starts with rewriting. I was worried about embarrassing myself and others (not to speak of the fact that I am basically a private person). Yet as a writer, a writer with cancer, I seemed to have no choice in the matter. So I began to record how I was feeling and what was happening all around me. I soon got the idea that it might be useful to others if I could publish my journal in monthly installments in a national magazine. My literary agent agreed, and within days, *Self* became the first magazine ever to publish such a series.

The response was more than gratifying, and letters and comments came in each month of the year my journal ran. And after a while I became brave enough to see that there should be a book as well, and I expanded certain parts of the journal as it was originally published. *Living in the Lightning* is the result.

A CANCER JOURNAL

November 27, 1995

Late this afternoon I was diagnosed with cancer. I learned that I had a form of non-Hodgkin's lymphoma called "malt," for "mucosa-associated lymphoid tissue." My oncologist, J. Gregory Mears, M.D., said that mine "was not a bad story," because my tumors were "indolent," slow-growing. Not a bad story? Doesn't just about everyone know that non-Hodgkin's lymphoma is incurable? I have incurable cancer. Jackie Kennedy Onassis recently died from the same disease. What was good about any of this? Dr. Mears's words were hard to take in, but my husband, Christopher, and I strained to listen carefully.

There are two basic types of lymphoma, cancers of the body's immune network: Hodgkin's and non-Hodgkin's. Cell structure determines which is which. The microscope had shown mine to be one of ten forms of non-

Hodgkin's lymphoma. Mine was low grade. When I brought up Jackie Onassis, Dr. Mears said that her lymphoma had been very fast-growing and was completely different from my disease.

"Malts," a fairly recently defined medical entity, are tumors that grow outside the lymphatic system, in odd places like the gastrointestinal tract and lungs (or even, heaven forbid, in the tear ducts). I have a visible five-and-a-half-inch indolent tumor sitting in the fatty tissue of my lower back, and CAT scans and MRIs taken over the past week also revealed a smaller tumor in my thoracic region, lesions at the base of my lungs, as well as two tiny tumors in the pelvic lymph nodes themselves. A test had revealed that there was no bone marrow involvement, the only good news as far as I am concerned.

Although my cancer is incurable, it is "manageable," Dr. Mears says. "Think of it as a chronic disease." I must now regard myself as having a condition like, say, diabetes. Dr. Mears emphasizes that none of my symptoms is "terribly threatening," that he does not see "grave" danger to my life "now," and that "the picture is not black." There is a relatively new chemotherapy drug called fludarabine that has melted away tumors like mine. Dr. Mears says that the B cells in my tumor "have forgotten how to die," and that this drug "makes the cells learn to die again." (B cells are one of two types of white blood cells—or lymphocytes—crucial to the body's immune response. T cells are the other type.)

I had a hint of what was coming on November 22,

when a biopsy revealed "lymphoid cells where they shouldn't be," as a pathologist put it. The next day was Thanksgiving and my husband and I and our seventeen-year-old son, Noah, a high school senior, somehow managed to crawl through it. We had dinner at a neighbor's house. Our twenty-six-year-old daughter, Rachel, a graduate school student in California, was spending the holiday with friends in San Francisco. She was worried and comforting at the same time, phoning often throughout the day and night. Noah, the family computer expert, printed out pages and pages of important news about lymphoma from the Internet. He gave them to me only after my diagnosis was certain, and then only the pages concerning non-Hodgkin's.

I'd forgotten that November 22 was the anniversary of John Kennedy's murder, and was only reminded of it when I watched the late news on television. I remember once saying that I'd never, ever, forget what happened to our country on November 22, 1963, but now cancer had driven it right out of my mind.

When I first heard the news of the extent of my illness, I was stoic. But when Christopher and I drove home from the hospital, I wailed. The cry seemed pitiful, like that of a stranded wild animal. It was a wail that I had heard from my body only one other time: when I was ready to push Rachel into the world.

My life will never be the same again, I know this to be true, but I will have to learn that this is cancer in the 1990s, and that cancer, too, will never be the same again.

November 28, 1995

I've often said that my friends are my family, and it's true, although I should say they are my extended family because that is even truer. Christopher, Rachel, and Noah are so *there* it's like I'm never alone, even though I know I will have moments of feeling alone. Actually, I've always believed that everyone *is* alone, and it's just good luck that now and then others can "see" us.

I have also always held that we must accept dying as part of living. Now I am to be tested. I know that by thinking about death, as I have these last few days, I am not being morbid, but rather, I am making myself— trying to keep myself—more alive. Acceptance of death is a way to keep growing. I truly believe this, yet I can't find the strength to share these thoughts with anyone right now.

Rachel asks if I am scared. No, I say, I'm sad. Noah asks very few questions. He keeps searching the Internet for more information.

My main tumor is in the center of my lower back. "Why there?" I ask myself. Is this the same as asking, "Why me?" I hope not. I'm not someone who asks that question.

November 29, 1995

I've bought dozens of books already, and have made a trip to the library as well. I'm thinking of joining a support group, too. I want to know and to confront everything. I want to know all the facts about my condition all the time. I hope my oncologist can "survive" me.

A book called *After Cancer: A Guide to Your New Life*, by Wendy Schlessel Harpham, M.D., contains what should be my mantra: "The important question is not whether you have negative thoughts, but what you do with them. Negative thoughts reveal your fears and concerns, not your beliefs." The bookstore didn't have Harpham's first book, *Diagnosis: Cancer: Your Guide Through the First Few Months*, so I have read how to cope with the aftermath of treatment before I have read how to cope with the first few months. Do I always have to do things differently? Even my large tumor is unusual, so unusual that two months before my diagnosis one doctor mistook it for a lipoma, a benign fatty tumor, and another doctor who looked at it about two years ago when it was still a minor bump, or rise in my skin, said it was just the way I was built: "It's your posture."

Which leads me to another "mantra" from Dr. Harpham: "Laugh every day." I could write a book on this particular advice. Christopher and I have been practicing it for thirty years. When we can laugh at or about a serious situation, we always know we can, will, or already have come through it. Sometimes we're the only ones who laugh, but that's okay: it's the secret of our life together and as a family. On a drive to postpone Christopher's jury duty at the Bronx County courthouse before meeting Dr. Mears for the first time, I kept seeing signs in the Spanish supermarkets along the Grand

Concourse that advertised "MALTA: 4 For $1." What is Malta? I kept asking my husband. He lapsed into a schtick about its possible meanings that had me laughing hysterically all the way to the hospital. When Dr. Mears said my lymphoma was called malt, we could barely suppress our laughter. I remembered how I fell into waves of uncontrollable laughter when I stood next to my father's coffin thirty years ago. I had been ashamed until I was later told that such a response was not uncommon. Dr. Mears had noticed our amusement—did he think we were crazy?—and Christopher then told him about our "malta" adventure on the way to see him. He laughed, too, at the coincidence. I later discovered that malta is a nonalcoholic beer. It soon became the name for my tumors.

"Laugh every day."

November 30, 1995

Dr. Mears is "on the fence" about my treatment, which will be chemotherapy because I have too many sites involved to have surgery or radiation. We could watch and wait for a while, he says, since I have hardly any complaints of pain or discomfort. I read that this option, "watchful waiting," is controversial even though studies have shown that it does not affect a patient's long-term survival. "We intervene when there is a problem, like a blockage." I am sure that my lower back tumor is growing. But the scans contradict me, confirming that it is the same size it was over the summer. I am suddenly aware of every sound my body makes. My neck hurts. I get frequent headaches. (I am sure this is stress.) My lower back hurts when I stand too long. After all, the tumor is pressing on muscle. My body itches. Is it one of the distressing symptoms of lymphoma, meaning my condition could be worsening, or is it my cats, the blankets, or simply the "winter itches"? I have no fevers or night sweats, other ominous signs. I know a lot about this. I have been turned into a permanent second-year medical student by the extensive research I did for my latest book.

"We're not in bad shape here," is Dr. Mears's own mantra. I am having trouble hearing him. He says that there's a lot of research activity going on. "In two years we might be looking at a different picture," he continues. After all, fludarabine (a type of chemotherapy called an antimetabolite that starves cancer cells by tricking them into accepting the wrong building elements, as well as blocking the formation of the right ones) is only five years old. What might be discovered in the next five years, by 2001? Why is it so hard to listen to this good news? Will I be alive in 2001? The average survival for malt lymphoma is anywhere from five to ten years, although patients have lived for thirty years. I am in stage four, the most serious level, although this "staging" does not sound the same doomsday note for lymphoma as it does for other cancers, like ovarian or breast cancer. I think about my former sister-in-law, Nancy, with fourth-stage ovarian cancer, who is more alive than ever four years after her "doomsday" diagnosis of two years. The new miracle drug, Taxol, is responsible for keeping her cancer under control. She still has cancer throughout her body, she tells me, yet she feels fine and looks fine—radiant in a flowing wig she likes better than her real hair—and has even fallen in love. The man knows about her condition.

December 1, 1995

At one point today, I turned on the car radio at full blast to drown out my crying. Driving alone, I had been thinking about why I cleaned out my study so thoroughly (and aggressively) a while back. Did I have some premonition of my cancer? I threw out copies of old (bad) poems, as well as my attempts at novel writing (very bad). But I also got rid of some things I wish I hadn't thrown away—files from my days as a poet/teacher with The New York State Poets-in-the-Schools organization. I see that I was too hasty in some of my decisions. From now on, I must try to think and rethink such matters.

December 2, 1995

I did it again. I forgot a landmark date. It wasn't until nine tonight when we were out to dinner on the Upper West Side with some friends that I realized that I hadn't acknowledged my newborn Rebecca's death nineteen years ago today. Does this mean my cancer diagnosis has completely taken over my brain?

December 3, 1995

I have to give a talk about *The Girl Who Died Twice* tonight. I haven't done much preparation, although I have outlined the topics I want to discuss. I am hoping the lecture will take on a life of its own.

December 5, 1995

I raced around Chanukah and Christmas shopping today. I wanted to keep moving and stop thinking, and I finished more than half of my list.

December 8, 1995

I'm just about finished with the holiday shopping. I have never done it all so early.

December 24, 1995

Despite everything, it was a "sweet" Christmas Eve, as one of my relatives put it.

I have been sleeping poorly, and waking up a lot during the night.

December 28, 1995

A doctor friend suggests that I seek a second opinion even though I am extremely happy with my oncologist, who is with Columbia-Presbyterian Medical Center in upper Manhattan, just a few miles from my house. "Ten years down the pike you might ask yourself if you took the right path," my friend argues. "It's not a bad idea to check things out now." He knows of a young doctor in Boston who is an expert in lymphoma. My husband, Christopher, and I decide to drive there for a consultation.

The night before our trip I feel a deep sadness. In my mind I go down to a place I have never been to before. I face death as closely as I ever have, I think, and perhaps in doing so, some anxiety lifts. Strange.

The Boston doctor, Michael Grossbard, is brilliant. He should be at the hospital where Dr. Mears works. They could make an inspired team. Meanwhile, I am relieved to hear the same mantra: malt is "treatable, treatable, treatable!" I also hear how malts have "a tendency to go to the lungs." So are my "lesions" definitely lymphoma? Probably, but it isn't worth doing an invasive biopsy to find out. Once treatment begins, a CAT scan will show if they've grown or disappeared. And treatment should begin right away, Dr. Grossbard insists. During the past few weeks I have felt definite signs of change: my lower back aches more than before; my buttocks often throb like an annoying toothache; shooting pains sometimes go down my thighs. My legs feel weak. This is new and real. I am in touch with my body. A heating pad and Advil help. I have not yet told Dr. Mears of these changes, but I will at my next appointment. He already knows that I am 99 percent in favor of beginning treatment anyway, as is Christopher. The doctor in Boston is concerned that the tumor could invade my spinal cord. "Don't leave it sitting. It's as likely to grow inward as lengthwise."

Fludarabine is not any better than some standard chemotherapy treatments, I am told by Dr. Grossbard. It's a good drug insofar as it will not cause hair loss or nausea, but it will depress my immune system for about a year. Dr. Mears has already warned me of this, and has also told me of the other drug choices. Indeed, Dr. Grossbard does not believe that fludarabine is the best choice for me. As it happens, Dr. Grossbard has participated in a study in which patients received three infusions of fludarabine a week instead of five. The results were the same. "There was a complete response," he says. He also gave his patients the antibiotic Bactrim three times a week to ward off infections. Out of twelve patients, only one—a woman with very advanced disease—came down with an infection, one that landed her in the hospital for a few days.

It's actually up to me to decide. *Cancer in the nineties.* What about patients who are not as medically sophisticated as I think I am? How can they decide? For that matter, how can I?

January 10, 1996

Dr. Mears believes that chemotherapy should start at once when he hears about the changes in my condition, and he seems agreeable to trying the Boston way. My first treatment is scheduled for Tuesday, January 16.

A friend tells me that I speak so matter-of-factly about

my cancer. "I don't know how else to do it," I tell Beth, and it's true. Is there really something unusual about this approach? Another friend tells Christopher I have "great courage." This isn't courage at all; it's just plain common sense. And this friend wouldn't think I was so courageous if he saw me tonight. I'm in a crying rage over the smallest things. I bought the wrong kitty litter. The kitchen floor is overwaxed. The outside of the house needs painting. And I'm in a frenzy over the cost of my cancer treatments, even though my health benefits are excellent. But all that money spent to curb a disease that will kill me anyway, unless of course something else does first. Like my high blood pressure. The silent killer. Christopher hates when I talk like this, although he listens. He always listens.

I remember the feeling of *relief*—of all things—that I experienced shortly after my diagnosis. So this is how I'm going to die, I thought. One great mystery solved. Something not to have to worry about. So that's what's in store for me. I'm going to be dying of cancer. Like my father in 1964. Only this is 1996, and everything about the disease has been transformed, I try to remind myself.

What helped me get through all the tests and probes I have had to endure is the knowledge I acquired in writing my recent book. Medical education in American hospitals was transformed because of the controversy arising out of the death in 1984 of eighteen-year-old Libby Zion. The long and tiring hours worked by interns and residents was questioned across the country, and New York

State created an eighty-hour-per-week limit, with no more than twenty-four consecutive hours on duty. (Eventually these regulations were incorporated into the internal medical section of The American Medical Association's Graduate Medical Education Directory.) In addition, I uncovered what I called the best-kept secret in hospitals, and the dirtiest little secret in medical education: the closed-order book. The closed-order book means that unlicensed interns can write medical orders without obtaining permission from anyone in the hospital. They don't need always clearance from resident supervisors or senior doctors, because, as I wrote: "This was how one learned to be a doctor. . . . and from California to New York, all across America, the closed-order book, and the lack of minute-to-minute supervision of interns it encouraged, was the law of the land." When—or if—I were hospitalized at some future point, I would be able to understand the medical hierarchy.

I also had discovered a great deal about the routines and politics of everyday hospital life. So when a radiology aide had difficulty while injecting me with dye and told me my vein was the cause of the trouble, I knew she was blaming me to cover up her incompetence, a not uncommon response among hospital workers. (The dye going in felt very similar to the feeling one gets from those seat warmers in cars!) Later, a nurse in the oncology department had no trouble at all with that same vein when she drew blood. Patients have to speak out! I didn't to the radiology aide because I have decided to pick my battles carefully, and that one seemed too tiny. But is it? What about what it represents in terms of hospital care?

During another CAT scan where I first had to drink a huge quantity of liquid, during a pause I asked to use the bathroom. " 'They' don't like you to get up," the aide said. "But why?" I asked. "I'm not hooked up to anything." She asked if I could wait until the test was over. "How long will that be?" I asked. "Twelve minutes," she answered. "No," I said, "I need to use the bathroom NOW." And I did. Later I asked if I could see the pictures. "She usually doesn't let you," I was told. Never one always to accept no, I walked into the "computer room," anyway, smiled politely, and said I just wanted a peek at my interior, and that I was a writer. "I know," the radiologist said amicably. I was pleased, but more pleased to see the pictures, even though they were baffling. But still, the inside of my body, as clear as rain.

January 11, 1996

I am a cancer patient, and will be for the rest of my life. But I must learn to think of myself as a survivor. Indeed, Dr. Wendy Schlessel Harpham writes in her book *After Cancer* that "cancer survivors include those who have just been diagnosed." Harpham also mentions something else helpful: "You know and accept all the truths, but you do not let yourself think about them all the time." I aspire to such a state, but at the moment I am not even close, even though I fully acknowledge the reality of my condition. But I cannot stop thinking about it all the time.

A close friend who is also a writer reminds me today that "our most precious possession as writers—our imagination—is actually my enemy in dealing with my disease. "You must not imagine anything about it," he counsels. "You must rely only on the facts." I try to remember this advice, especially late at night when my thoughts often drift out of control.

In a phone call, I tell my former sister-in-law, Nancy, about my cancer, and that I will begin treatment in a few days. Her positively bubbly spirit has always amazed me, but I get depressed and angry when she confides that "I have never read anything about cancer, and I have never asked my doctor any questions." I decide she must be joking—some joke—but she isn't. "We're going to have to find a way to communicate without words," I tell her, ashamed of the sarcasm in my voice. I realize that in the past whenever we have spoken of her ovarian cancer it has been in a vague, unclear way. I went along because I didn't want to be too intrusive. But now that I have cancer I am wondering if all along her luminous spirit has been just a form of denial. Why does it matter if this is what it takes to get her through a terrible illness? Where is my compassion?

Everyone reacts to disaster in a different way. After all, it was only recently, I remind myself, that I understood the miserable black humor of Mel Brooks's musical extravaganza, "Springtime for Hitler," in his famous movie,

The Producers. When I first heard the song, I was appalled by its lack of taste. I was therefore shocked to hear myself humming the tune the other day. Where did it come from, and why did it burst forth now? I hated it! What was happening to me? Finally I decided that my unconscious was "speaking" to me, and saying that some things are so horrible that the only way out of them is through the darkest form of humor. I soon found myself fantasizing about a glitzy event to be called The Cancer Follies. All of us survivors would tap and sing our way toward— toward what?—a remission? a cure? Did I suddenly lack shame, and dignity, too? Was I going nuts?

What senselessness often accompanies anguish. I remembered that during the painful bone marrow aspiration (a deep, searing pain) two months ago, I told Dr. Mears that I was trying to think of how much I used to enjoy beef marrow on warm rye bread as a snack. He was bemused, I think. I asked him a lot of questions during the procedure—as a way of keeping my mind off the discomfort. (I had first asked him if my talking distracted him, and he said no, it didn't.) I asked him about his background, his education, his marriage—I was so pleased when he said that his wife is a doctor, too. His mother died of breast cancer. He said, "I remember coming home for Christmas from med school, and the silver wasn't polished. Then I knew she was really sick." I liked him for telling me that. I brought him a copy of *The Girl Who Died Twice* inscribed "Here's to a *long, long* journey together." Most people want their trips to the doctor to eventually stop. Not me. When mine stop, perhaps I too will have stopped.

Very briefly, I felt a "Why me?" trying to come out today. But I wouldn't let it. It's bad enough that I felt it *trying* to come out.

January 12, 1996

Ever since my diagnosis, my extended family—my friends—bring a kind of comfort I almost didn't know existed. "The love Marilyn and I feel for you is the love we feel for each other," Hugh tells me today. Two other friends "demanded" to see me at once. "You look so well," they all reassured me. And this is true. In fact, I decide I have never looked better in my life. Yet I have cancer. Another visit by some neighbors had felt like a condolence call. I wonder if other people will begin to treat me differently.

In private, I begin to squeak. I kid you not. From time to time I find myself letting out little—well—squawky squeaks. Finally my husband asks me why I am doing that: "What's that little sound I hear?" I tell him perfectly straight-faced that it's a cell going out of control. My son breaks up. How can I want to make him—me—anyone— laugh about cancer? I am supposed to be a serious person. I'm definitely going insane. Or I'm desperately groping for a way to deal with the news of my cancer. I decide that it will take at least six months to get used to the idea that I have an incurable disease.

Some time last week my daughter initiated a reconciliation with a beloved brother-in-law. I cry with joy that old hurts can be forgiven, and better yet, never spoken of again. I read somewhere—I can't recall where—that letting go of grievances is good for cancer patients, survivors. (I still have trouble with that term, *survivor*. Why?) I think that whatever I read said that keeping some grievances also makes sense. I decide to hold on to several, the residue of unreliable, unrealistic relationships. There is a fine clarity and glowing satisfaction that comes with these decisions.

Some friends are now calling every day. Some lost friends start reappearing. Acquaintances I have admired from a distance suddenly call and express concern. I learn something important from all of these calls—medical advice, psychological advice —after all, for all of my life I have been told that I am a good listener. I take everything in, but follow only what my instincts (and oncologist) believe is a constructive path.

January 14, 1996

An informal support group is beginning to spring up as a result of friends and neighbors learning about my cancer. My literary agent, Lynn, asks the writer and publisher Michael Korda if I can read the manuscript of his new book, *Man-to-Man*, on his struggle with prostate cancer. He sends it. It is an astonishing book—brutally honest and brave. It makes me cry. "The truth, no matter how it looks, is the only route to healing," I write to him. He agrees, and answers that "the truth, however brutal, is the most important means of survival."

I had met Barbara Barrie, the actress, at a New Year's Day party. She is a colon cancer survivor. She begins to send me chapters from her moving book-in-progress, which will be published sometime in 1997. We share the same oncologist and she gives me tips on my chemotherapy treatment, which will begin in two days. I am haunted by her words: "Your cancer will bring you gifts."

Meanwhile, I obsess about what to wear to chemo. During one of my rounds of buying and borrowing library books on cancer, I remember flipping through one that said you should always look nice or even dress up when going for treatments. I put that book right back on the shelf, thinking, what kind of person needs such superficial advice! Well, clearly, me, because I have to confess that it is the advice I think about the most at this point. Obviously, I put the book back quickly (how I wish I could now give its author credit) because I was ashamed to admit how much that advice was meant for me. After all, shopping is my only hobby, a fact I share only rarely with others. Like many people, I also find shopping a way to deal with stress, and conversely, when I find myself obsessing about what to wear someplace I know that stress is present.

Now I begin to realize why I always wear my favorite outfits to my doctor's appointments and why I am always sure to have freshly washed hair on those days. I definitely want to look "nice," and I am keeping my anxiety in check. Do I also want not to look sick?

January 15, 1996

My first chemotherapy session—appointment? injection? I don't even know what to call it, which strikes me as downright ridiculous—begins at ten A.M. tomorrow. I realize that my concern over what to call it is a symptom of the anxiety that has been building up in me for the past several days.

My son, Noah, gives me a letter he has printed out from the Internet. I actually get chills. My God, I am benefiting from personal information delivered from cyberspace. (That I can't get it for myself yet is another story, one that will be resolved soon, I hope.) A woman who calls herself "Grannybarb" addresses "Dear All" from her website, saying that she has been through two rounds of fludarabine therapy (the drug I will begin tomorrow), and finds it "very user friendly." I could hug "Grannybarb." She reports feeling queasy for only an hour or so after treatment. I am reassured by this report, and wish I could call her (by telephone!) and ask her some questions right now.

Instead, I call my friend Dalma and we discuss what I should wear to chemo. As always, these fashion conversations that we often have are relaxing, amusing, and beneficial. I decide to wear my long brown velvet skirt with a particularly well fitting long-sleeved black tee shirt.

Dalma, a writer, has great style and shopping know-how. She introduced me to M.A.C cosmetics when I went to Boston for my second-opinion consultation, and made sure I wore "Media" nail polish, the red-black color of the moment. Now she says that I must use a pearlized gloss over my regular lipstick. These so-called "superficial" details really help ease my anxiety. "A person must try to worry about things that aren't important so he won't worry too much about things that are," I read somewhere long ago.

January 16, 1996

The room where I am to get my treatment is large, sunny, and airy. It has grayish-green walls trimmed with a band of Egyptian-like patterns, and a peach tiled floor. It is decorated with paintings of rolling hills and rocky beaches, and art deco lamps that give off a pale light.

I am not particularly nervous, which surprises me. Nonetheless, I begin to wonder what I'm doing here, because strangely, the discomfort in my back and legs has almost become an acceptable companion. I don't look or feel "sick," so why do I have to join the eleven or so other people I see sitting in comfortable-looking pastel-colored lounge chairs scattered around the room? In fact, as I look around more carefully I see that most of these people also don't look sick.

My friend Shelly, whom I nicknamed "Bell" twenty years ago, had called me at nine to say that she polished the silver bell earrings I gave her for her fortieth birthday. "It's my way of sending you good luck, and love," she said. My neighbor Carol, whom I call "Earth Mother," insisted that I use her family's car service to take me back and forth to the hospital on all my chemotherapy days. It is now a welcome gift that I accepted only reluctantly at first because it seemed so extravagant. But it gives me one less thing to think about, especially since I wanted to come to the treatments alone. I had everything planned. After I had the required blood test in the oncology lab, I would go to the treatment room, sit down, listen to 101.9 jazz radio on my earphones, and write in my journal. The time would fly.

I am introduced to Allison Kimberg, one of four oncology nurses. She directs me to an empty chair. Her voice is warm and soothing. I look around the room some more. Is the woman wearing a maroon tee shirt and matching leggings who is reading *Money* magazine a patient or a visitor? What about the neatly coiffed ash-blond woman in pressed jeans and a well-tailored jacket sitting next to a gray-haired man in a navy pinstriped double-breasted suit? Or the bronze-skinned woman with fuscia lipstick wearing a floppy black felt hat with a large pink rose on it? I see that they are all attached to IV lines. What kind of place is this? *This is cancer in the nineties.*

Allison hooks me up to an IV drip that is giving me saline solution only. We make small talk while awaiting word on my white-blood-cell count, and she tells me that she and her co-workers have been together for almost a decade. I am impressed. "We're like sisters," she says. I ask her if they ever fight. "All the time," she says, laughing.

If my count is good, the fludarabine will begin. I've read that a cubic millimeter of normal blood usually contains 4,000 to 10,000 leukocytes, or white blood cells. Dr. Mears says he wouldn't treat someone with a count below 3,000—and says if a count was 1,500, he'd be "worried." My count comes back 8,500. I know that it will drop as I remain on chemotherapy, putting me at risk for infections, although I am taking the antibiotic drug Bactrim three times a week.

I had asked Dr. Mears if I could see the fludarabine bottle at each infusion, and he had agreed to this. Ever since a cancer patient at the Dana Farber Cancer Institute in Boston had died in 1994 after receiving the wrong chemo drug, I, like many other people, have been wary. My own research when writing *The Girl Who Died Twice* had already dramatized for me the importance of checking and rechecking medications thoroughly. Anyone in the health care profession can make a mistake. When possible, patients must try to look out for their own welfare; medical care must become a joint effort between the patient and the hospital staff. Gone are the days of "maternal" or "paternal" doctors: patients can no longer act like children, even though their illnesses often make them want to regress. But as we approach the year 2000, everything in medicine is changing and becoming more complicated, and patients, more than ever, must be alert and sensitive to what is happening around them.

Allison starts the drip, and lets me keep the fludara-bine bottle as a souvenir. She thinks it is a strange request, I know, and warns me not to put it in my "regular" trash. I have no intention of ever throwing it out, because somehow I feel that this tiny glass bottle on the shelf above my desk at home will act as a constant reminder to me of where I am (in life) and what I have to do to continue living.

January 17, 1996

I arrive for my second chemo at 10:15 A.M., and this time all the chairs are filled, so I must wait for a vacancy. Allison gives me a friendly smile. Yesterday the whole procedure took no more than forty-five minutes—it's not bad at all. No ill effects so far, either. Not even Granny-barb's queasiness. One more treatment tomorrow and then it's over for the month. I'm going to be having four to six such thrice-weekly cycles. Dr. Mears believes we'll see "a good response" in just one or two of those cycles. I have already learned that "response" is a medical code word for tumor shrinkage, and is used by oncologists to sound more upbeat, as the word *remission* does, and, of course, the word *cured*.

Speaking of words, there are some that have been giving me pause lately: Fight. Battle. War. I cringe when I read phrases like "the war on cancer," or hear people refer to my "battle" with cancer or say I am such a "fighter." Why do I cringe? Shouldn't I feel some pride? I think I have this unusual reaction simply because the killing field is not level. I wish people realized that at this point my lymphoma knows more about me than I know about it. It knows exactly how and where to go within my body, but I can't track it or ever get rid of it completely. So, in a way it's a losing battle from the start. But that doesn't mean I'm not a player. I soon decide that what I can do is fight—do battle with—the symptoms of my disease. It's a subtle difference, I suppose, yet somehow more acceptable. Even though the fludarabine can't kill the individual cancer cells that are roaming my lymphatic system, it can shrink or destroy the tumors created by those rogue cells, thus buying me time. I can win that "war." I have a tentative truce with these "embattled" words.

My wait turns out to be only five minutes. This time the needle that infuses the chemo into my bloodstream hurts my hand a bit, and Allison adjusts it, saying it is pressing on the vein. We talk about a concert she attended last night. I look around the room. I don't see many faces from yesterday. An elderly man sitting three chairs away from me starts coughing violently, and one of the nurses draws a curtain around the area where he is sitting. (I notice that all the areas where there are chairs have gray-print curtains pushed off to one side.) I can hear the man retching noisily. This, too, is cancer in the nineties, I have to remind myself this morning. I think of the telephone conversation last night with my elderly mother. Despite her being healthy and very active, I had considered not telling her about my cancer because of family burdens she already carries. But when she asked me how I was one day, I blurted out the news. Last night she asked me if the people in chemo looked "very sick." I told her that most did not, and that if we met them on the street we'd never know that they were struggling with cancer. But she persisted. "Do any look really bad?" "Yes," I finally said, one or two looked "very bad." "Poor souls," she remarked, ending the discussion.

Allison checks on how I'm doing. She says my drip is slower than it was yesterday. I ask her why. "Perhaps it's the vein I used," she answers in a calm, confident voice. She moves off to help another patient. 101.9 radio tells me that it will be fifty degrees tomorrow. Spring in January. I look around the room some more. I notice three women wearing various types of silk or cotton turbans. I notice that the woman who yesterday wore the black floppy hat with a rose on it is today wearing a suede turban. A companion puts a blanket around her. Several other patients are also snuggled in blankets. I didn't notice any blankets yesterday. A nurse whose name is Eileen opens the curtains around the man who had been vomiting. His face looks peaceful now, but his color is ashen. His exposed arms look pale. The arms of a woman next to him are so white they look like candles, or pieces of plastic. This effect is accentuated by the bright red nail polish on her very long fingernails.

January 18, 1996

Infusion number three. I am very weary today. I am also constantly on the verge of tears. While grocery shopping late yesterday afternoon, I actually had to leave the store and go to my car to lie down.

Allison had told me that I might have headaches (I did) and would probably feel "very tired." I do. I know from my reading that this tiredness will be both acute and cumulative. Dr. Mears told me that, too, of course. I feel no nausea.

The tiredness is more flulike than anything else. And my eyes are constantly teary. I'm not crying, but almost. I suppose that in time I will learn to recognize this as a symptom of fatigue and will adjust. But right now, I feel very strange and very sad (not exactly depressed). The pain in my back, buttocks, and thighs is constant; no position seems right or comfortable. Is this my new life?

I think of the book Christopher was reading a while back, a book by an M.I.T. professor about the effects of computers on literature and life. Somehow the subject of computer sex came up in a conversation, and my husband said, "Maybe that's what I'll do when you are gone—I could never replace you." I said, "You shouldn't be looking for a replacement, but something else. Maybe a thirty-six-year-old will be enamored of a gray-haired ole man." We were silent. Had the discussion gone too far? "I wouldn't want that," Christopher finally said; "I'd rather be alone." Although it was liberating to be able to talk so freely, I didn't want to say anything else.

January 22, 1996

I speak to Faith, an old friend who has mesothelioma, a rare form of cancer of the lining of the abdomen. Last spring, 40 percent of her tumors were removed by surgery; now she and her doctor are doing "watchful waiting." She is also doing "complementary" medicine—vitamin drips, supplements, herbs. "My immune system is in great shape," she tells me.

I have read a lot on such complementary medicine, and after a discussion with Dr. Mears, I have decided to add just one to my daily vitamin usage: astragalus, a Chinese herb that supposedly boosts immunity. Although this herb is described in great detail in all the books I have read on the subject, hardly anyone I know uses it, or has heard of it, even the friends who call me regularly with their own discoveries.

At dinner last evening, Dalma said I looked "pale." This afternoon, after I demanded honesty, Christopher said I looked "pasty- faced." I am tired. It's four days post fludarabine cycle number one.

I feel grateful that Zerina, our part-time (but live-in) housekeeper postponed her three-month trip to Zimbabwe in order to help out. The other family she works for was also grateful she's staying, because they have two young children Zerina helps care for.

January 31, 1996

Dr. Mears reports that my original tumor, the big one on my lower back, has shrunk half an inch already. He says he is "thrilled." So am I, although I can't feel any difference when I touch my back. I am always checking, hoping I will notice the shrinkage. I decide it must be like trying to watch a bud burst into flower. You can never manage to see it happening before your eyes.

Last night Christopher and I went to Ikea in New Jersey to buy a rug for our living room. We found just the right one, as I knew we would—a Southwestern design in muted pinks, blues, and greens. Afterward we sat in the store's café having a snack (a bag of Swedish fish for me). I became very weepy over the thought that some other woman might live in my house after I died. Christopher just listened to me, of course, and then quietly told me that if I died before he did, he'd live in the house alone, and if he remarried, he'd buy a new house. I liked hearing this—not only because it seemed real—but because such truth-telling heals.

February 12, 1996

Chemo month number two, and I'm sitting here on day one like an old-timer, listening to 101.9 jazz radio and writing in my journal. Christopher has accompanied me today, and waits in a comfortable chair next to me reading a biography of the poet W. H. Auden. My white blood count of 5,100 is still in the normal range 4,000–10,000).

This morning as I was dressing I became aware for the very first time that the tumor in my lower back is definitely flatter. I almost can't believe it. I rubbed my hand over it to be sure I wasn't dreaming. No, I wasn't.

Dr. Mears told me that the fludarabine carries on its work all the time, not just during the treatment. Praise be! It is, of course, starving my cancer cells by setting up a sort of hoax. (Other types of chemotherapies stop or slow down cell growth, or disrupt cell division.) So all month long, fludarabine has been performing its treachery on my DNA, and in just a few short weeks, there are positive results. (Fludarabine, in use for only a few years, evidently plays very little havoc on the DNA of normal cells, although there is always the danger that it might, which is why many patients fear chemotherapy. The FDA approved fludarabine in 1991 for use only in the treatment of chronic lymphocytic leukemia; however, it is common for oncologists to expand the usage of most single-indicated drugs. According to Dr. Mears, fludarabine "is still being investigated in different cancer settings.")

Oddly enough, I think that at this point Dr. Mears might be more worried about my high blood pressure than my cancer. He wants me to buy a home monitor; in fact, for the past week I have been dealing with various heath product companies that are listed in my insurance booklet. According to the regulations, the cost is covered if I have a doctor's order, which I do. Still, one company insists on payment upfront (by me) and another says it doesn't understand why it is listed because it is not part of the plan. A third company says it is sure it can accommodate me and will look into the matter and call me back. It doesn't. When I call a second time, it has no record of me. I am sure my blood pressure must be rising. A friend suggests I forget the insurance route and just buy a home monitor at my local pharmacy—"it's only a hundred bucks," she says nonchalantly—and sheer frustration almost leads me down that path. But I am saved by Thuyen Nguyen, who came to America from Vietnam in 1975. He works in the office that oversees my health insurance program, one that has three different components (it's not as complicated as it sounds). Miraculously—to me— "T-N," as this gentle man likes to be known, makes a single call, and the red tape is unsnarled.

February 14, 1996

For the past three days, I have been aware of a bronchial type of chest pain. It's not horrible, and feels a little like the beginning of the flu. I had felt the pain very slightly a month ago, but Dr. Mears didn't seem concerned when I told him about it. Now it is also accompanied by a cough. I worry about the lesions on my lungs that were seen in my first CAT scan.

The man sitting across from me looks like a living corpse. I see that in addition to chemo, he is receiving blood. I wish I knew all about these people in here today. Who are they? How are they coping? What chemo are they on, and for what kind of cancer? Allison is discreet, but does tell me that two people in the room are also on fludarabine.

It's a snowy Valentine's Day. As I look out the window,

I see that the sun is pushing through the clouds. Everyone is hoping the snow will melt soon. Oddly, the bright sun peeking through makes me sad. Here I am—infusion number three, the last one for the second month; my "malta" is shrinking; I look well; the discomfort in my back and legs has lessened—and I'm sad. I soon realize that this sadness is simply more of my mourning for a cancer-free body. Even during a remission, I will be thinking about the cancer cells and when they will start forming tumors again. I'll be thinking about this forever. Terminal worry. Still, I decide on a new goal: to have a day—or part of a day at first—when I do not think about my cancer at all. I know it will be possible.

The receptionist in the chemo room is wearing a giant red-felt heart pinned to the back of her sweater. Allison calls out that she's watching my line and I'm almost finished. "This is the best part of my day, being here. I love people," she says as she removes the needle from my hand.

I think of what Dr. Michael Grossbard, the Boston oncologist I saw for a second opinion, told me: "Try not to let this illness change your life."

It's my Valentine's Day plan.

February 26, 1996

"It's time to do some CAT scans to see what is going on inside," Dr. Mears tells me. He thinks that my chest pain and cough are most likely a side effect of the fludarabine. (The lesions can't be totally ruled out as the source until I have the new scans.) When I was reading the literature that accompanied the fludarabine bottle, I saw that in two reported trials of the drug on 133 patients, 10 percent reported a cough in the first test, and 44 percent reported a cough in the second test. At first, Allison had been reluctant to give me this literature, thinking it might frighten me. It didn't, even though it lists a total of some seventy possible side effects. *Seventy!* I compulsively looked up every single one in my medical dictionary so I could be armed with the facts. I find that knowing them strengthens my resolve to fight my symptoms.

I have developed a persistent feeling of pins and needles in my arms, hands, and fingers (also, my nails are flaking and peeling). I have difficulty picking up small items, like change or buttons. I am tired all the time now. It is a tiredness not helped by napping (although I now sleep nine or ten hours a night). I feel drained.

Still, my family and I have pretty much kept to our normal schedule of work, chores, and going out to dinner or the movies with friends. We are all fairly independent, so no one relies on me to do certain set things. Still, Christopher and Noah took their cues from me—pitching in more when they sensed I needed it, like offering to pick up groceries at the supermarket, even though they know I enjoy all such errands. (It's true.)

Dr. Mears says that the tingliness and finger clumsiness is nerve damage from the chemotherapy. "Damage?"

Christopher, the book critic, asks him during my appointment; "Damage?" Dr. Mears looks at my husband thoughtfully. "Well, okay, nerve *injury*," he amends, because it is not necessarily permanent, as the word *damage* implies. I also had a brief spell of mouth sores the first month, but they disappeared very quickly. All in all, I consider these side effects minimal, a nuisance, like having a mouse in the kitchen.

February 29, 1996

I have the CAT scans taken today at a place in New Jersey that bills the entire cost to a new insurance option that recently became available to my family. The office is professional enough, yet somehow makes me feel like a second-class citizen. Do I miss a hospital setting? In any case, I'm going to hand-deliver a set of the pictures to Dr. Mears and his own radiology department, and receive their analysis of the films as well.

March 11, 1996

Today is the first day of my third month of chemotherapy. My white blood count is 5,200. It is also the day I learn the results of my CAT scans. Christopher is now on jury duty, and cannot come with me.

The oncology department's waiting room is not crowded. Dr. Mears greets me with a smile. "There's a wonderful regression of your disease," he says when we reach his examining room. The lesions on my lungs are gone! (So the cough is a side effect of the chemo.) The lymphoma in my upper thoracic area is "90 percent gone." The swollen pelvic nodes have disappeared. What about my main—the original—tumor? "There's a real good response, but it's not all gone. There's still abnormality there," he says quietly. Actually, I knew this already. When I saw the doctor in New Jersey looking at my films I had asked him to measure that tumor, and his calculations had indicated some shrinkage, but not an enormous (or satisfying) amount. Still, Dr. Mears seems happy enough. "After two more treatments, we'll reassess things," he says. "We might consider adding radiation if we are left only with the lower back problem—to mop things up. We'll wait and see."

Cancer requires a lot of patience.

March 13, 1996

During my appointment with Dr. Mears two days ago he used a term that I didn't pick up on right away. Actually, it is commonplace for a patient not to hear what the doctor says until days or weeks after he or she has said it. (Sometimes patients don't hear the message at all.) In my case, after Dr. Mears made a reference to the continuing "abnormality" in my lower back, he had added that he "didn't know if this was new disease or scar tissue." It was not until I got home and reported this to my husband, Christopher, that a light bulb came on. New disease? Did that mean I had two different kinds of cancer—one on which the fludarabine worked, and the other on which it didn't? How could that be? What was going on?

I was scared and confused, and knew that my befuddlement was caused partly because my patient advocate (Christopher) had not been able to accompany me due to his being on jury duty. If he had been with me I know that he would have picked up on that "new disease" in a flash.

But there was also another facet involved. During my appointment, Dr. Mears had seemed mildly distracted, as if some heavy weight was on him that afternoon. I felt that something was wrong, and asked him if he was okay. He said that it had been a bad week. He looked distressed when he said this, so I decided not to push, and the discussion returned to me. But I spent some time worrying about him.

On the way to chemo (day three of month number three) this morning, when I stopped by Dr. Mears's office to ask Karen, his secretary, whether I could have a word with him either before or after my treatment, Dr. Mears was standing by the doorway, and so I made my request directly to him. He said we could talk now. As we walked into a treatment room, I told him how I had been upset by his using the term "new disease" and added that I had been a "bad" patient for not dealing with it at the time. Was the fludarabine not working in some spots? He quickly replied that he had misspoken, and that he meant to say "persistent" disease, not "new" disease. There was no new disease. "The important thing to remember," he emphasized, "is that the volume of the original tumor *has* diminished." Then he asked why in the world I would call myself a bad patient. I told him that my friend Shelly ("Bell") had asked the same thing. I said that she thought that the only reason I hadn't asked for clarification was because I was too busy taking care of the doctor. Dr. Mears looked surprised, and then said warmly, "You were." He also said that I had been the only patient that day to notice that something was troubling him, and then he told me what it was.

Not only was he enmeshed in office politics (no place is more political than a major teaching hospital!) but he was anxious about a talk on the Reformation that he had agreed to deliver at his church in Connecticut on Sunday. "What do I know about the Reformation?" he asked, and I realized that the preciseness and clear intelligence he used in his practice of medicine was now being challenged because he was entering a field where he was not an expert. Who wouldn't be nervous? I, myself, wasn't even sure exactly what the Reformation was. Partly for that reason, but mostly because I was curious about the kind of talk he would deliver, I asked if I could see a copy. He reluctantly agreed.

Bell, a psychoanalyst, had remarked to me that the topic of patients "caring" for their doctors was an important—and neglected—one. She wondered if any studies had been done on the subject. I, too, wonder. All I know is that medicine has to be a two-way street. It really does.

41

As we approach the 2000s, and insurance plans and medical plans develop faster and faster and faster, patients—especially cancer patients—have to be very involved in their medical care (it's practically my theme song). And patients need to show compassion for their doctors. Naturally, an inattentive, careless, or trivializing doctor deserves little or no understanding. But I think that because medicine is moving to new places, patients now have to go places they never dreamed they'd have to: inside the heart and mind of their doctors. It will do wonders for everyone's health.

March 14, 1996

All during chemo yesterday, I—a non-observant Jew—was obsessed with a young Hasidic couple. They seemed to me to be in their late teens or early twenties. The young woman, wan, yet beautiful, in a long cotton dress, was receiving chemo, and her black-suited husband and a colleague were circling around her. After a while, some older people—relatives?—entered the circle. Their presence was so large that it seemed to me as if they were the only ones in the room. At one point I noticed that the young husband was sitting still, reading, and his entourage was quietly surveying the scene. I asked Allison, my nurse, if she could find out what the husband was reading, but I didn't expect an answer (even though by now she was getting used to my nosiness). So I was delighted when Allison whispered to me that she thought he was reading the Torah. Reading the Torah in chemo! Why did that strike me as completely incongruous? The holy Torah! As I looked up from my journal and continued staring at this pious family (did I have no shame?) I saw the husband stand and move to a corner of the room. He had such a baby face. Why did his wife have to have cancer? Would she be able to have children? He took something small and flat out of his pocket. A religious object? Some mystical relic? No, a cellular phone! He talked for quite a while, his colleague standing close by. They were both very animated and excited. The young husband's expression looked sincere, yet mysterious. To whom was he talking? Shortly afterward, everyone gathered to leave quickly (the wife, too), and I became aware of a great void in the room. I missed this family. I had even felt slightly envious of their religious devotion. For a while, I had forgotten how tired I felt, how depleted.

March 25, 1996

An appointment with Dr. Mears today. Barbara had one, too, and we decided to arrive a little early so we could have time to talk. We are a one-on-one support network.

Actually, a while back I explored the possibility of joining some sort of official support group, but my search proved disappointing. For instance, when I called the New York chapter of the American Cancer Society to ask if there was a support group for non-Hodgkin's lymphoma patients, the person who answered my call made me repeat my disease twice and then explain what it was. "It's a form of cancer," I said. The person answered, "We don't have groups for that." I then dialed Cancer Care, Inc., and a person told me that I'd have to make an appointment with a social worker. "But, why?" I asked. "All I want is a list of your support groups. Can't you just send one to me?" But the person reacted crossly, "Do you want to see a social worker or not?" I wondered how I got caught in such a miserable spider web. Was I dying? Had I committed a crime? Finally, I said angrily, "No, no, thank you," and hung up.

I should have known better. After all, hasn't it been in the past five years or so that New York City's once-dependable telephone operators not only began to get snippy at simple requests, but also began to make mistakes? And haven't drivers been using the left lane on highways as a slow lane and the right lane as a passing one for just as long? Public behavior is changing. Why should the cancer world be immune? Later I asked Allison about a possible group at the hospital and she said the only ones she knew of were for breast cancer and prostate cancer survivors. But she took my request seriously. Then I decided to try the Internet again. I e-mailed Grannybarb some questions about other people on fludarabine. She just referred me to her home page, which I had already read. I suppose I could start my own group at the hospital, by putting up signs in the oncology waiting room and the chemo room. But I don't really want to do that. I've decided I'd rather put my energy in other places—like thinking of a new book project. I have enough support from my family and friends.

March 26, 1996

Yesterday Dr. Mears had admitted that I might not see a complete disappearance of my lower back tumor. I was concerned, to say the least. I was actually expecting all my symptoms to vanish, at least for a while. So, I might have to live without this happening: the original tumor is smaller, flatter, but still there under the surface. During our discussion, Dr. Mears reminded me that "we're on track for an excellent response." But, still, where exactly am I going? (One thing I know is that my white blood count is dropping—on schedule—it's now 3,900, slightly below normal.)

I've got to get off the emotional roller coaster. Good news. Bad news. Fair news. Highs. Lows. This is one ride I'm not taking, even though all the books I have read suggest that I will have to coast along. No. I won't.

I've made a decision to try to regard all information about my cancer as neutral news—not good news, not bad news, just continuing—flowing—information about my condition.

Am I just playing with my mind? I don't think so. The only good news I could really hear is that a cure has been discovered for malt lymphoma. So short of that, I will now try to hear all reports of tumor size, tumor shrinkage, even tumor appearance—and of course, disappearance—as straight, neutral information. I think I can handle that ride.

April 5, 1996

Friends are people who listen to your agonies and dreams. After I was diagnosed with cancer, I blurted out to Dalma and Marilyn something basically inconsequential: a wish for something that has been beyond my reach all of my life, yet has remained an ardent fantasy. I said, "One thing I'm going to do now is get myself that black Armani jacket." Of course, such a purchase was still out of the question, what with my steadily increasing medical expenses, not to speak of my son's upcoming college tuition. Yet dreams give one courage, it is said, especially in the face of danger. So I kept on dreaming.

A few weeks later, my husband and I had dinner at Shun Lee West in New York City with Dalma and Richard and Marilyn and Hugh. During drinks, Dalma suddenly turned to me and said, "We have a little something for you." She took a small, oyster-colored shopping bag from her purse. I saw the words Giorgio Armani written across the front of it, and my breath stopped. "Is this a trick?" I asked. "No, it's not," Dalma said, smiling. Marilyn and Hugh were smiling, too. I reached into the bag and pulled out an elegant card, opened it, and among the many words on it I saw only these: "a jacket." My hands were trembling. I looked around the crowded restaurant. I looked down. I looked at my husband. I burst into tears. My friends had bought me an Armani jacket.

"Oh my God," I finally said. I kept staring at the gift certificate. No one had ever done anything like this for me. I was the one who gave gifts. How in the world could I accept this? It was far, far too extravagant. "We knew you'd feel that way," Dalma said tenderly. "But it's all paid for so there's nothing you can do about it except pick out exactly the jacket you want."

"Now she'll have nothing to live for," my husband quipped, as we all hugged and kissed and cried. My family of friends.

April 8, 1996

Chemo month number four begins today. I see Dr. Mears beforehand, and receive two pieces of news. (I'm putting my neutral-news approach to the test.) First, my blood pressure is dropping, thanks to medication I am now taking thrice weekly. Second, an ache on my right side that I've been experiencing for the past few weeks is not cancer pain, but is caused by chronic gallbladder disease. "There's no lymphoma on your gallbladder," Dr. Mears says. In fact, a scan has shown a gallstone, but until recently there had been no symptoms. Dr. Mears suggests I take an ultrasound test to check further, and I will get one in two weeks when I have a new set of CAT scans taken. (On top of everything else, cancer consumes a lot of time!) I might need to have my gallbladder removed at some point after I'm finished with chemotherapy. When I express apprehension about going through such surgery with lymphoma, Dr. Mears says, perfectly straight-faced, "Why? You're healthy." I look at him as though he were a crazy relative. He forms a slightly mischievous smile. To an oncologist, a cancer patient who is active, working, and relatively free of pain and infection is, well, "healthy." Of course, I know he means healthy in the sense of fit, not free of illness. But how I wish he meant the latter.

I have to wait about fifteen minutes today for a chair. The chemo room is buzzing with activity. I don't see many familiar faces.

As Allison hooks me up to my fludarabine, Dr. Mears enters the room and hands me a copy of his talk on the Reformation. (I had reminded him to earlier.) "Don't judge the grammar," he says. "Oh, I will," I say teasingly. He answers, smiling, "That's what I'm afraid of." As he leaves the room, I start to read it. This talk is just like his doctoring! Knowledgeable, exact, and down-to-earth. I had wanted to read it to find out more about him, and I did. I also learned a lot about the Reformation. I even found myself puzzling over the Episcopalian position on humility because of something he wrote about religious adoration. Maybe I'll discuss this with him at some point, but probably not.

I settle in with my journal and 101.9 jazz radio. Even though my earphones pretty much filter out sounds in the room, they don't filter out what happens next. A loud, piercing alarm goes off. Oddly, no one moves. No one. The alarm shrieks and shrieks, and life in the chemo room goes on as usual. "Is it for real?" I ask Allison. "I don't know," she answers. A few moments later she tells me that it is a smoke alarm, and that everything is all right. But what if it hadn't been? How much time would it have taken to disengage everyone from their drugs? Could I have just pulled the needle out myself and run? Even stranger than everyone's remaining so passive during the alarm was the fact that, as I realized, I didn't want to run. I wanted to stay where I was. I did not want the flow of fludarabine into my bloodstream to stop, even for a fire.

April 9, 1996

This morning there are some familiar faces. The woman with the black floppy hat with a red rose is today wearing a white bowler hat trimmed with three roses— one red, one white, and one pink. She looks radiant in a white suit and shiny black leather boots. How sick is she? Very, I had supposed, from the way she huddled under her blanket last month. Yet today she looks as healthy as a newborn.

Before I turn my radio on, I become aware of a pleasant-looking woman in her early or mid-seventies sitting across from me. She is crying that the needle hurts. "They don't believe me," she says over and over, between sobs, to her husband, who looks helpless. Allison hurries over to help.

"I think she's having trouble with her foot," I hear some-one say. Allison offers to remove the woman's sneaker. The woman calms down, although when I next look I notice that her sneaker is still on. Probably she only had a panic attack. I become aware that my own needle is hurting. I tell Allison and she makes some adjustments.

One thing I've noticed lately is that I think less often about my having cancer. Five months have now passed since my diagnosis. Am I learning to get along with my disease? I think that my adjusting to my cancer is one of the reasons I write in my journal less often than I used to. I no longer do it daily, except during chemo week. So perhaps when the urge to write everything down goes away—although I seriously doubt that this will ever hap-pen—I will have adjusted fully to my new life.

April 23, 1996

I'm to have my second set of scans taken today at the place in Englewood, New Jersey that makes me wish I were having the pictures taken at the hospital. My atti-tude seems so ridiculous because all the technicians are first-rate, and Dr. Mears has said that the previous films were perfect. But something about the place makes me uncomfortable. Could it be that I'm anxious about what the pictures will show?

"Bell" says she wants to meet me there so she can try to understand my complaints. "It's perfectly profes-sional," she comments after looking the place over, "but also slightly seedy. I wouldn't like to be here, either." I somehow feel better after she says that. I've got three scans and an ultrasound ahead of me. My insurance pays the entire cost. After "Bell" is told by a technician that, because of the radiation emissions, her being in the room is not a great idea, she decides to go off grocery shopping. We'll meet up again when I'm finished. I notice that one of the technicians has an award tacked on the wall proclaiming her an Employee of the Year according to some national organization.

After forcing myself to drink the special liquid that will enhance the pictures (a contrast dye is also injected into a vein in my arm), I lie on a hard plastic table that can be moved in and out of the open donut-shaped CAT scanner. The procedure does not make me feel at all claustrophobic, the way an MRI can. An MRI is enclosed (although some newer ones are open on the sides). But when I had an MRI (at the hospital) I felt as if I were being pressed into a toothpaste tube. Several years ago, Noah had to have an MRI when his eye was injured at school, and he reminded me to ask for a pillow and music, two things he had been offered. I did, and it helped. Also, some basic instinct took over and I closed my eyes during the entire test. I opened them only when the technician told me there was one minute left. I didn't like at all what I saw: the tight, tight sides of a narrow white tube that enveloped my body. I was glad I had kept my eyes shut.

During my CAT scan, I think of how Rachel, my

twenty-six-year-old daughter, figures out how I am feeling by asking me whether or not I am writing. "Have you started your new book?" she asks. When I say no, she is concerned. "But I *am* writing my journal," I reassure her. She doesn't think of this as my "real" work because, well, she wants me to be far, far away from my cancer. I try to explain to her that I am not quite ready to tackle "Fundamental Women," my working title for a book about the lives of right-wing women (I haven't even picked the ones I plan to write about). Yet until I do, I know Rachel will be frustrated. Still, I like how my feminism has shaped hers: a woman is healthy only when she is working at her passion. A few days ago I told her that I felt stirrings of wanting to get moving on the book idea, and she said, "Oh, good, that means you are learning to live with your cancer."

April 24, 1996

Yesterday afternoon I dropped the scans off at Dr. Mears's office. I called him at six this evening to get a report. He said that he hadn't gotten a chance to take them to the radiology department because a twenty-year-old woman with leukemia had suffered cardiac arrest, and was being resuscitated "as we speak." He also mentioned another dire emergency. "So please forgive me," he said softly. He said to call tomorrow. "I don't know how you do this job," I said to him toward the end of our conversation. "I don't either," he answered.

April 26, 1996

A meeting kept me from calling Dr. Mears yesterday at six P.M., so I called this evening. Since I now considered all news to be neutral, letting a day go by didn't seem unusual. However, the news he gave me made me realize that I have been playing mind games after all, and that my neutral news routine isn't working. Not only do I long for good news, but I need to know if news is not good, and I long for the freedom to feel sad about bad news. So I'm back on the roller coaster. Some rides just take you where you don't want to go.

The ultrasound of my gallbladder showed that I have not one, but two gallstones. The dull ache on my side persists. "We can't operate while you are doing chemo," Dr. Mears reiterates. The upper thoracic tumor "might be gone," he says. As for my original, lower back tumor—my main "malta"—it's only "somewhat smaller." And, Dr. Mears adds, "truthfully it's not a lot smaller." He had warned me exactly one month ago, on March 26, that I might not see its complete disappearance. Still, I feel sad. So, as well as not being able to sustain my straight, neutral news approach, I now seem in danger of becoming the kind of boring patient who keeps on despairing over news that has already been explained by the doctor.

April 27, 1996

During a pause in my conversation with Dr. Mears last evening, I had asked about the young girl with leukemia.

LIVING IN THE LIGHTNING

"Did she make it?" Dr. Mears was silent for a moment. "No," he finally said. "She died." Then he told me that shortly before her death, she had delivered a one-pound, ten-ounce, premature baby, and, he added, "the baby is doing fine." I don't know what in the world possessed me to ask the next question, but I did. "Is the girl who died by any chance the beautiful young Hasidic woman I recently saw in chemo?" Dr. Mears seemed startled by my asking this, and I quickly added, "I don't mean to intrude on the family's privacy, but I liked watching them. I think I even borrowed some of their piousness for a little while." Dr. Mears then told me that yes, the girl who had died was the young Hasidic woman. "They are a remarkable family," he said.

My grief for them made me forget my own worries and complaints, and I fell asleep that night thinking of the baby, born of a child who died in the sweetness of her life.

May 1, 1996

I read in *The New York Times* this morning that a study at the University of Iowa College of Medicine revealed that women between the ages of fifty-five and sixty-nine who consumed more than thirty-eight portions of red meat each month were twice as likely to develop non-Hodgkin's lymphoma as those who ate fewer than twenty-two portions. Fortunately, my family only eats red meat four or five times a month, and usually less. But the part of the article that haunted me the most was this line: "The incidence of the disease [non-Hodgkin's lymphoma] has risen about 75 percent since the early 1970s for reasons that are unclear."

Is it something in the environment? Pesticides? Chemicals? Food additives? Food supplements and/or vitamins? What is out there, or inside the body, that causes this cancer, and has made me one of the 52,700 Americans diagnosed with non-Hodgkin's lymphoma this year?

And what about my children? Are the risks greater for them, not only because of possible environmental factors, but because of me, and of course, their grandfather (my father) and many of his ten brothers and sisters, who also died of cancer? Somehow I feel confident that the reasons for the increase in non-Hodgkin's lymphoma will be found. And there are so many new drugs—and treatment approaches—on the horizon. Cancer can be controlled, if not cured. I find this immensely reassuring when thinking about what the future holds for Rachel and Noah.

May 6, 1996

Day one of chemo month number five, and I acted as if it were my first. While getting dressed in the morning, I stood in my closet for what seemed like an hour because I couldn't decide what to pick out. Why am I so nervous about my treatment after all this time? Finally I had to call Dalma, and she helped me decide what to wear (new long black skirt, old brown tee shirt). I'm ashamed of my idiotic indecision today. But I think I know what caused it: treatments number five and six are the ones that can put my white blood count way under the norm. My count right before my infusion today was 4,100, just a tiny bit above normal. So what awaits me after two more cycles? When my immune system is "knocked out" (as Michael Grossbard, M.D., the Boston doctor I consulted, put it) will my body be overrun with infections of one sort or another despite my taking Bactrim?

I can't help thinking of Nancy, with late-stage ovarian cancer. Two weeks ago she was hospitalized with a high fever caused by a severe kidney infection (she has a mass on one of her kidneys that is causing a blockage) and almost didn't make it because her immune system is so weak from her chemotherapy treatments. She doesn't understand why this is happening to her. Her denial about her condition is extreme; in fact, in a recent phone call she even told me that she attributes her "doing well" these last few years to her "total denial." Her verve is still dazzling. "My dating pattern hasn't changed at all," she told me exactly one day after being released from the hospital. Where does she get the strength? The man she was in love with a few months ago is no longer in her life. Now she has decided not to tell her dates that she has cancer. "I'm doing what's best for me. These guys don't tell me the truth," she said. During our most recent phone conversation, a week before she was to reenter the hospital for surgery to remove her mass, she told me, "I can beat the odds. I can't wait to walk briskly."

Maybe most people would find my way of dealing with cancer just as curious. A few weeks ago I practically forced Dr. Mears to tell me exactly how I would die eventually. He resisted, but finally gave in. He told me that "pneumonia is the most common way for lymphoma patients to die," and said that right before death I would be "bedridden, weak, and depleted." I have found that knowing this has given me renewed strength to fight my disease. I need to know everything, everything. Nancy needs to know nothing. "I know nothing. I don't care," she told me.

May 7, 1996

Yesterday while waiting to see Dr. Mears before my fludarabine infusion, I became aware of a noisy couple in the oncology waiting room. Usually I like to eavesdrop on conversations, but this one was making me irritable because of a combination of their slow, depressed-sounding drawls and their inane political comments. I decided to put on my earphones and listen to 101.9. But I could still hear them. So I raised the volume until my eardrums were tingling. This was the first time I behaved like that at the hospital, and I am now wondering if this was really caused by that couple, or by something else I didn't want to hear.

I talk to Allison today about the death of the young Hasidic girl. She is very sorry about it. "Why did she die?" I stupidly ask. "Because of her disease," Allison answers me patiently, explaining further, "She had an infection as a result of her treatment. This is all part of the disease."

Allison later tells me that "everyone in the hospital deals differently with death. But we tend to remember 'presences,' so no one is really gone."

May 8, 1996

The last infusion of the month. All week I have positively dreaded the needle going in, something that normally hasn't bothered me very much. Allison explains that the needle hurts more now because my veins are so scarred.

Today I am sitting next to one of the two chairs that have small televisions attached to them. They're for people who are having all-day infusions. The TV to my right is turned on softly to a soap opera, but the woman in the chair is asleep, covered snugly by a white blanket. She is receiving a blood transfusion along with her chemo. I look over at her from time to time to see if her eyes have opened. She sleeps on. I turn my attention to a woman who is using the only bed in the room as a desk. She has moved a straight-back chair up close and is working away on a laptop computer. Papers are strewn all around. She looks very businesslike, and if I hadn't seen the chemo bottle and line next to her, I might have taken her for a healthy hospital employee. The woman sitting next to me stirs, opens her eyes briefly, but then falls back to sleep. I watch her and soon spot a familiar object lying on the windowsill next to her. It's the black floppy hat with a red rose! I hadn't recognized the woman, and I worry that her condition has deteriorated because she is sleeping so much. What must I be thinking! Everyone with cancer deteriorates sooner or later. I begin to feel very tired and stop writing in my journal and turn off my radio. I close my eyes, and think, dear God, all I am doing here is postponing death, and for how long until some horrible infection kills me? I'm just sitting here waiting to die. But, I say to myself, we are all "waiting" to die. Allison stops by and says my drip is too slow. She makes some minor adjustments to speed it up.

What finally lifts me out of the doldrums is reminding myself what Allison said to me two days ago. "You look great." I thanked her, and told her I felt great. And I do. Some people have said I've never looked better in my life. I haven't used a heating pad on my back in weeks. I use Advil less and less. Even the gallbladder pain seems to have subsided. I've started to use my treadmill again (some unwelcome pounds are showing up). I am adjusting to being tired and have learned to pace myself appropriately. But I still have not had a complete day of not thinking about my cancer.

Allison tells me about a man who was in treatment a few days ago who exclaimed, "Why am I here? I feel great." It's the great chemo puzzle. Have cancer. Get chemo. Chemo holds cancer at bay (or cures it in some cases). Begin to feel like you don't have cancer. But you do. (And will always need treatment of one sort or another.)

Anyway, the real puzzle for patients is this: how to feel when you don't feel you have cancer.

May 10, 1996

While waiting for Dr. Mears in a treatment room during my last appointment, I noticed my file had been placed by a nurse in a black plastic holder attached to the outside of the door. I removed it, and started to read it. I didn't expect to find anything new in my record since Dr. Mears has given me (at my request) copies of everything. But as I was riffling through all the papers, I spied a letter I hadn't seen before. It was addressed to my internist, and was a summary of my cancer treatment so far. Page two contained this phrase: "Discussions have pointed out that the goal of treatment is palliative and not curative . . . "

The word "palliative" threw me. *Palliative: "Relieving or soothing the symptoms of a disease or disorder without effecting a cure."*

I had to sit down in the only chair in the room. What a fool I must be—talking all the time about how the truth is the best way to deal with cancer when a word that I've seen a dozen times in all the books I've accumulated, a word that accurately describes my treatment, this single word sends me into despair. What is the matter with me? I seem not to be able to take my own medicine.

When Dr. Mears walked into the treatment room and saw me reading my file he commented, "Pretty boring, huh?" I mumbled something inane, probably, "uhhmm."

But during my exam I said, "I don't know what's the matter with me today. Seeing the word 'palliative' in your letter to Dr. Tenenbaum makes me so miserable." He looked at me quizzically, and said calmly, "But I've never used the word *cure* with you. Never." I looked up at him. "Of course you haven't. I've understood my situation from day one. I know there's no cure for my lymphoma, and this fact is burned into my brain. I just think that seeing that word 'palliative' typed out like that—so bold, so raw—has made a small difference to me." Dr. Mears nodded sympathetically.

The power of the printed word.

May 19, 1996

I learned recently that a very close friend has been diagnosed with non-Hodgkin's lymphoma. My first reaction was idiotic: had she caught it from me? My second reaction was a little more rational: what could be in the atmosphere that has given us both this disease? I thought about this a lot, particularly because my friend, Diana, understands food better than anyone I know, and has been saying for years that things don't taste as they used to. Have we both unwittingly been eating some terrible additives? We both do a lot of reading: is there something in the ink, the paper, the glue? What about television? Computers? Microwave ovens? Plastic containers? Lotions? Lipsticks? Dry cleaning? Gasoline?

My friend Diana is ninety and it is hard for her to be

subjected to as many tests as she has had to be. Still, for the most part her experience at her hospital has been a good one, and her doctors and technicians have been kind to her, listening to her requests and making her comfortable. But when radiation became the treatment decided upon, she was told to report to the hospital for a half-hour fitting for a shield to protect the part of her body that was not going to receive the radiation. This fitting took more than two hours, and my friend, who leads an orderly, highly scheduled life, was treated rudely, even cruelly, when she complained—not about the time involved—but about the fact that the bun and hairpins in her hair were causing her pain because of the position she was lying in. No one suggested she let her hair down, and by the time she thought of it herself, she was coldly instructed to remain still. "I was treated like a piece of meat," she said. She was angry, frustrated, and felt demeaned.

As her radiation treatments proceed, she is learning. When told she needed a weekly blood test, she insisted that the technicians in her own doctor's office do the blood drawing. "They don't hurt me," she said. After much discussion at the hospital, this was permitted. A small but critical triumph for my elderly friend. The more she speaks up, the better she—and her treatment—will be. For the most part, the elderly are not treated with respect in our health-care system. Indeed, many people even react with horror—with horror!—when they hear that my friend is being treated for her cancer at all! Why bother at her age? they seem to be saying. But my friend wants to go on living—just as I do—and has important business to finish. Besides, she is more productive at ninety than some people I know half her age. Radiation gives her, as she says, "a fighting chance. I don't like taking death without fighting a little."

Cancer, of course, doesn't care how old a person is.

May 24, 1996

I decide to check in with Dr. Michael Grossbard, the doctor at Massachusetts General Hospital whom I saw for a second opinion six months ago. He had asked me to keep in touch (Dr. Mears sent him an interim report), and with my sixth (and final, for now) cycle of fludarabine coming up in two weeks, it seems like the right time for another consultation. Besides, my son will be in Cambridge for the next four years, and keeping in touch with an oncologist nearby when we visit him also seems like a good idea.

Dr. Grossbard, as before, is very straightforward. (This quality endeared him to me forever when I asked him why he went to Yale instead of Harvard for medical school after being an undergraduate at the latter and he quipped, "They rejected me. But I'm over it now!") He has seen all of my radiology reports and two of my scans, and, unlike Dr. Mears, puts a number on the actual shrinkage of my main "malta." "There's been a 20 percent reduction," he says. Even though I already know this tumor has not shrunk as much as we had hoped, the small number he uses jolts me. I expected to hear 50, or even 60 percent. "Why only 20 percent?" I ask him, but I mean by my question, Why does it feel as if the number should be bigger—or is bigger—and why hasn't the fludarabine done a better job in that spot? "There's still a lot of bulk there," he says, "and I'm sure there's a substantial amount of disease, too." It's not just scar tissue. Again he tells me that he is concerned that the tumor could compress my spinal cord. He thinks I should consider skipping my sixth treatment of fludarabine, see a radiation expert right away, and also consider using a different type of chemotherapy, a combination of several drugs that Dr. Mears had told me about. These drugs—Cytoxin with vincristine or chlorambucil (alkylating agents that disrupt cell division)—have been around for over twenty years. They cause hair loss, nausea, and vomiting. The addition of the steroid prednisone, which enhances the brew, often causes weight gain. All at once I understand why interns and residents have a slang term for a consult. They call it an "insult." Although Dr. Grossbard was neither taunting me nor offending me, his advice was like a verbal jab. I didn't expect to hear what I heard.

At my most recent appointment with Dr. Mears, when he told me about the minimal change in my lower back tumor, I had asked about switching chemos, and he had said no. Or at least I think he said no. When I first began treatment, he and I discussed all the alkylating drugs, and decided not to use any of them. For one thing, Cytoxin has been known to cause secondary leukemia. But today I am more concerned that Dr. Mears and Dr. Grossbard seem to be so far apart in their approach to my treatment than I am troubled by Dr. Grossbard's actual recommendations. Still, I decide not to call Dr. Mears about the dilemma, but rather to wait and talk to him about it in person in two weeks. Besides, in my own mind, I know I am going to go ahead with fludarabine number six, and proceed with Dr. Mears's plan to have a PET, or Positron Emission Tomography scan, soon afterward. During this scan, radioactive ingredients will be injected into my bloodstream to measure metabolic activity, and the scan's three-dimensional pictures may be able to pick up clusters of cancer cells in my body. This test is the most advanced nuclear technology available. "It's an intellectual exercise," Dr. Mears said, explaining that it "could show us where you stand with your lymphoma." The PET scan, recently available for patient use, is very expensive, but the hospital will accept my 80 percent insurance coverage as payment in full. Although Dr. Grossbard is less sanguine than Dr. Mears about the scan's usefulness for my purposes, he says it is "harmless."

Yes, cancer in the approaching millennium involves new technologies and new treatments, but it also involves new etiquette. On the one hand there are Dr. Grossbard's ideas, which I want, and on the other hand, there are my hands-on oncologist's ideas, which, of course, I also want. I feel comfortable and can make a satisfactory decision when they are close in their opinions. I liked that Dr. Mears agreed to give me the fludarabine Dr. Grossbard's way—three times a week instead of five. Still, I begin to feel the strain of managing them both. But this must be done, for it is the only way to able to decide what is the best treatment for me.

May 29, 1996

I call Dr. Mears today because I have been worrying about my treatment, and couldn't wait another week to learn his opinion of Dr. Grossbard's suggestions.

Even though I know it is my right as a patient to consult anyone I wish, I am afraid of hurting Dr. Mears's feelings because I like him so much. This is actually a silly way to feel, because he is a true professional, and welcomes outside opinions. Indeed, when he calls me back, he tells me that "what Dr. Grossbard said is not wrong," and "it's an individual preference." However, he does end up saying, "But our plan is good."

I agree. I feel it in my gut, too.

He goes on to say that it seems reasonable to get the "maximum benefits" from fludarabine, and therefore go for the full six cycles, and he reminds me that we took on Dr. Grossbard's "modified" plan. "You're taking 60 percent of what I normally give," he emphasizes.

Dr. Mears says that my lower back tumor "is not a threat to me," and for now, this must remain a difference of opinion with Dr. Grossbard. Dr. Mears also comments that often "scans are misleading," and says, firmly, "You're doing better than they indicate."

Difference of opinion or not, somehow I feel better after speaking with Dr. Mears. I'm following my gut feelings, too, and in doing this I'm probably doing one of the most important things that cancer patients can do for themselves.

June 3, 1996

Chemo month number six—the final one—began today. Christopher went with me. It was raining very hard, so he dropped me off in front of the hospital building before parking the car. Traffic was heavy and chaotic. I was already inside Atchley Pavilion when I glanced back through the glass doors and noticed a diminutive pregnant woman getting out of the passenger side of a car in the downpour. She seemed to be shaking her fist in my direction, and then I saw her scream at my husband, who had performed a clever, if rather aggressive, maneuver to get our car out of the street traffic and into the circular driveway of the building, thereby preventing the woman's husband from driving closer to the entrance. This maneuver clearly had enraged the woman and her husband, who was now also climbing out of their car. I felt sorry for Christopher but not enough to stay around and watch; actually, I also felt a little embarrassed, because I thought his driving had been slightly rude. So I went upstairs to get my blood test, and left him to deal with all the anger vibrating in the wet air.

Later, in the chemo room, Christopher whispered that I should look across the room. The angry man and his angry pregnant wife were sitting next to a very ill elderly woman who was receiving chemo. Just my luck. "Don't worry," Christopher said to me, "the man is trying hard not to notice us." Still, I felt very strange and conflicted, and my heart went out to them. No wonder they were so angry: their relative looked like a corpse. Would she be alive to welcome her grandchild?

Except at the very beginning, I have never gotten angry over my cancer or its treatment. First of all, who or what could I remain angry at? This is simply what life has given me and I quickly accepted it. And I am saying this as a person who gets angry at a lot of things, a lot of things. "You're a very angry person," I've been told by a wide assortment of people most of my life. But I'm not angry about my cancer. A friend remarked to me that she was surprised that I was not in a rage all the time. But I'm not surprised. There's a saying—I've forgotten where it is from—that goes something like this: There are two things people should never be angry at: what they can help and what they cannot help.

Actually I was extremely sad after my treatment today, and realized it was because I was having a form of separation anxiety, of all things! My friend Hugh recently asked me if I was pleased to be finishing chemo this month, and I said no. He seemed upset until I explained that at least with the fludarabine I knew what to expect, more or less—but without it, I felt anxious about what would now be happening to my body. There are also so many unknowns to be faced about future treatments. I am frightened. Plain frightened.

I've been having tooth pain for the past three weeks, and finally saw the dentist four days ago. She thinks I'll need root canal work. Dr. Mears suggests I have it done this week, before my white blood count drops any fur-

ther (it was 3,700 today—4,000 is normal for a cancer patient). I told Christopher that I think I held off going to
the dentist for so long because it's an area of my medical
life I can control: I can decide when to seek treatment
and how much pain to endure. On the other hand, maybe
I didn't go out of fear that the pain would get even worse
(it did). As a child I was afraid of the dentist, a fear I over-
came as an adult. So I seem to be regressing. Will I be in
a fetal position by infusion number three on Wednesday?

June 4, 1996

My daughter, Rachel, home for a two-month newspaper internship that begins tomorrow, went with me to
chemo today. She has announced that if I need a chemo
that causes hair loss to shrink my lower back tumor further, she is planning to shave her head in solidarity. I tell
her no, no, but she is insistent.

"It's not that bad. It's just life," Rachel remarks after
Allison hooks me up to the fludarabine. "I like that there
are all classes of people here," she adds. She starts to read
a magazine. I'm writing in my journal. She says, "That
woman over there looks like she could be waiting for the
bus." Cancer in the nineties.

I like having her with me. Her involvement and understanding are very comforting. After the fludarabine has
been flowing for about ten minutes, I lean back in my
chair and close my eyes. A strong feeling of fatigue has
come over me. "Are you *very* tired, Mom?" Rachel asks.

"It's just a wave of tiredness, it's hard to explain," I tell her. "But it's not bad." Actually, I decide, it's a rush of fatigue. A new, and startling sensation.

Almost asleep, I decide that I am a coward. I dread having to lose my hair. I dread feeling sick. I dread gaining weight. (All are side effects from the more traditional chemotherapies.) I've been spoiled by fludarabine. I'm going to go through any additional chemo kicking and screaming, I bet. And I have to accept all this—including being a coward—if I want to live.

June 5, 1996

My former sister-in-law, Nancy, has an inoperable mass on her kidneys; her surgeon just opened her up, took a look, and closed her. The ovarian cancer has spread to her liver, too. I watch her with admiration and with awe, because she has begun to exhibit the most beautiful calmness I have ever seen in a terminally ill person. Her denial about her condition is gone when I talk to her today. Plain gone. This reversal—from abject denial to total acceptance—seems to have happened overnight. But it is real. She talks about her "remaining time." She told me that she is concentrating only on her relationships with her family and old friends. She has even set up a reunion with a long-lost cousin. She says that spiritually she feels "absolutely wonderful," and wishes she could say the same thing about her body. She is in pain most of the time. She is taking things a day at a time. Nonetheless, she is redesigning her apartment, is planning to buy herself a mink coat in August, and has already bought herself an $8,000 gold watch. "I'm fulfilling my dreams," she says.

But why would someone running out of time put most of her savings in an object that has more time than she does?

Maybe that's her point.

June 12, 1996

Today I have my PET scan at the Kreitchman Center at Columbia-Presbyterian Medical Center. According to a brochure given to me by the doctor who runs the program for the hospital (the only such clinical center in New York City), a PET scan "provides answers that no other technology is capable of providing."

"You'll be part of history," Dr. Mears said to me earlier. "I want to be," I answered, even though he also warned me that "we might find things that we won't know what to do about," like clusters of rogue lymphoid cells that have not yet formed solid tumors. Dr. Mears was concerned about whether I'd be able to accept such an indefinite situation. I said I thought I could handle it. I want to be involved with state-of-the-art medicine.

The PET technicians turn out to be extremely capable and kind, although the area where the actual test takes place (a few floors above a sleek reception suite) is pretty cramped and disorderly. I am escorted to a back room where privacy is minimal; in fact, another patient walks in twice without knocking or glancing my way. Here, in the only chair in the room—actually, I notice, this is primarily a storage facility—I receive an injection of radio-isotope tracer F-18, flurodeoxyglucose (FDG), to measure my body's metabolic activity. I am told I will have to wait about fifty minutes for this radioactive substance to be incorporated into my cells.

The machinery seems identical to that of a CAT scan. The test takes about an hour, and the results will be given to Dr. Mears within forty-eight hours.

June 17, 1996

An appointment with Dr. Mears today. He is running late because he has had to spend over an hour with a new patient. How can I get mad when he shows such compassion? Someday that could be me making other patients wait, and I hope they will be as accepting as I am.

While I am waiting, I learn that Dr. Mears has not yet received my PET scan report. When I catch sight of him in the corridor by the waiting room, I volunteer to try to round it up before my appointment. Christopher, who has come with me today to help me listen to the report, stays in the waiting room while I go over to the next building to see why 48 hours has stretched into 120 hours.

The receptionist at the PET center is very embarrassed, and in less than thirty minutes has the PET scan ready for me to deliver to Dr. Mears.

Dr. Mears reports that not surprisingly "there is disease activity in my lower back area." "But," he remarks somewhat delicately, "we might want to be happy that nothing else was picked up."

We are.

"It's a local problem now," Dr. Mears goes on, "and it doesn't make sense to hit you hard with more chemo in that one spot. We should save it for later in your life." Meanwhile, he believes that radiation therapy can eradicate the tumor, now that I'm officially a one-site cancer survivor. Looking at my state-of-the-art PET scan, he says that I've "achieved some good control with chemo. This is a picture of something that has gotten better."

With a little luck, after six weeks of daily radiation, I could be on my way to at least two years of no tumors at all.

It's called a remission: "*The period during which the symptoms of a disease abate or subside.*"

I'll call it a lull: "*A relatively calm interval, as in a storm.*"

July 8, 1996

Today Christopher and I met my radiation oncologist, Mary K. Hayes, M.D. Secretly I had hoped I wouldn't like her, the simple yet simple-minded reason being that I was beginning to get tired of giving my heart away to doctors. Was this the way it was going to be for the rest of my life? Doctor after doctor after doctor? My attitude seemed altogether unreasonable, especially since I didn't have that many doctors yet, and each new doctor could possibly provide a new clue to my illness. Still, out of anxiety—or perhaps even some strange form of restlessness—this was the way I was feeling just eight months after my diagnosis.

Dr. Hayes was both friendly and professional, and had a down-to-earth manner. So of course I liked her right away, and of course I was disappointed when she told us that she would be leaving Columbia-Presbyterian Medical Center next month to accept a job at New York Hospital (where she would be the clinical director of the department). I would therefore be the last patient she could take on in her present position.

We also met Dr. Lewis Smith, a genial fourth-year postgraduate resident who works with Dr. Hayes. He's my first resident since I began treatment at the hospital, and right away I began to wonder why there were no residents working in the medical oncology department, especially since I recently learned that Dr. Mears is the director of the oncology/hematology training program. I made a mental note to ask him about this at my next appointment.

The radiation oncology department is one floor below the hospital's basement, in what is called the tunnel. It is completely surrounded by thick layers of concrete and steel to protect the rest of the building (and the environment) from radioactive particles. I had been prepared for the atmosphere of a dank medieval dungeon (a description offered by someone radiated there four years earlier) but the area had been completely renovated and was bright and modern. Vases of fresh flowers abounded. It was hard to believe I was so far underground.

Both Drs. Smith and Hayes examined me. I know from my research on *The Girl Who Died Twice* that patients in teaching hospitals have to expect multiple exams—it's one of the ways residents learn to become experienced doctors. They "practice" on us. Dr. Smith was gentle and relaxed. I would have given him an A for thoroughness and demeanor.

Dr. Hayes called my malt lymphoma an "oddball" type of cancer. "They're odd players all around," she said in a peppy manner I found very soothing. But then she added something distressing: "We've always thought of malts as quiet, but recently we've begun to understand that this is not always true." Dr. Mears had said something similar months ago, but not quite in the same way. Or maybe I was now ready to take in this information, that malts can get aggressive, that malts can become fast-growing. As Dr. Hayes was talking to me about this, I almost, but not quite, longed for my short-lived all-news- is-neutral news approach.

Dr. Hayes reiterated that the PET scan had shown that I had "viable, residual disease." To the touch, my lower back tumor seemed like scar tissue. But it wasn't. She said that I'd probably need to receive between 3,000 to 4,500 centigray of radiation. ("gray," the name of a famous radiation doctor, is the term now used for one unit or "rad" of radiation.) These centigray will be electrons produced by an X-ray tube. The side effects would be minimal—

fatigue and "redness on your lower back." She stressed
that the goal would be "to continue to sterilize the area."
Such language began to make me feel as if I were part
of a military drill.

Before the treatment actually starts I am to have a
simulation session, which will use X-rays and a fluoro-
scope to pinpoint the area on my body that will be
treated, and then a "dosimetrist" will measure me to be
sure that this "field" is exact. I'll also be tattooed in five
tiny spots so that the field is marked permanently, and
can be identified for any future radiation planning. My
legs will be immobilized in a customized plastic mold to
assure that I stay in the same position for each treatment.
I'll also have a CAT scan—wearing my personalized
mold—to make sure that all the measurements are cor-
rect and accurate so that a radiation physicist can then cal-
culate the precise dose and angle necessary for my
treatment.

July 9, 1996

Naturally I've become obsessed with learning everything I can about radiation. I go on another book-buying
binge. I surf the Internet, though the material I find there
is too technical for me at this point. But in a newly pur-
chased book, *A Medical and Spiritual Guide to Living with
Cancer*, by William A. Fintel, M.D., and Gerald R.
McDermott, Ph.D, I not only read a clear, concise story
of a cell, but I also learn that radiation therapy uses col-

orless, odorless, and painless photons or electrons to eradicate cancer cells by damaging their DNA. True, normal cells are also damaged; however, when the treatments are spread out over several weeks, as mine will be, most normal cells can repair themselves. The cancer cells cannot.

July 10, 1996

Today is my son's eighteenth birthday. My husband and I and our daughter take him and a friend out to dinner at a steak restaurant he loves, and when the waiter brings my son a piece of his favorite cheesecake with a bright blue birthday candle stuck in the middle, I realize, to my astonishment, that I have not thought about cancer at all up to this point in the meal. Perhaps I'm beginning not to have to connect every event to thoughts of my disease. Perhaps I'm beginning to blend my dying into my living, or my living into my dying.

July 15, 1996

Today I learn that the radiation I will receive will come from a linear accelerator, a very high-powered X-ray machine. I am to have electrons aimed at my lower back tumor for less than a minute, five times a week for a month. The resident, Dr. Smith, told me that electrons have a negative charge and a fast energy buildup, and they "quickly drop off," unlike photons, which keep their energy long enough to pass through the entire body.

The simulation a few days ago was fairly effortless. I was a bit overwhelmed by the number of technicians moving in and out of the room, but, as I was told, the process requires absolute accuracy, and many different people double-check each other's work during the procedure. The person responsible for my tattoos evidently didn't have a checker, because I am now sporting a large black-and-blue mark around the tattoo on my right hip. Although Dr. Hayes downplayed it, Dr. Smith said he had never seen anything like it before, and joked that the technician responsible should lie low for a while. This person seems to have taken his advice. I noticed she looked away when she saw me arriving today, and I bet she continues to ignore me over the next month. Why couldn't she say a simple "I'm sorry" that would clear the air and help relieve her guilt; after all, the bruise is only ugly, not painful or bothersome, and I've been assured that it won't interfere with my radiation therapy.

July 17, 1996

Treatment number one began today, and at first it seemed like one of the most bizarre experiences of my life. I was lying on my stomach, with my head turned to the left side, on a flat black plastic and metal table that was raised about three and a half feet off the ground. The spacious room was lined with shelves holding dozens of plastic molds belonging to other patients. The cone of the linear accelerator hovered over my lower back. A special cloth that would intensify the dose of electrons was draped over my "field." I was told not to move. As two high-tech-looking red laser beams verified my position, the room seemed to take on an unearthly iridescent glow. I didn't know whether to be amazed or frightened. I remained still. I thought about what might happen if I suddenly decided to jump off the table. Would the machine stop? What would happen to me if the wrong part of my body was radiated as a result of an unforeseen leap? I wondered if the radiation technicians were doing everything right. Who hired them? What were their background and training? Had any patient ever jumped off the table before? I listened for sounds. There were none. I was alone in a sealed chamber. Eventually I realized that what I thought was some supernatural glow was actually the normal bright lights of the treatment room being turned back on after the room had been darkened for the lasers. I was so focused on the lighting that I didn't even hear the buzzing sound of the radiation, and only when a technician reentered the room did I figure out that my treatment must be over for the day.

July 21, 1996

When I was first told the routine—wait in the outer waiting room, go to the changing room when my name is called over the loudspeaker, change into a gown (actually it's more like a robe), put my clothes in a locker, lock the locker, and then go to the treatment area waiting room until I am escorted into the "bunker"—I questioned the need for a gown, especially a gown that left me exposed. "Wear two gowns, one going toward the front and one going back," I was told. "But why can't I do it like I did in the simulation?" I then asked. At that time, I had simply lowered the waistband of my long narrow skirt to my upper buttocks. "Well, that would be fine," I was told. "It's up to you."

Well, not wearing that short, silly gown made a lot of difference. Not having to change sped up the treatment time and made me feel less vulnerable. I wondered why other patients didn't do the same thing. Every single man and woman I passed in the corridor had those ridiculous gowns on, and they all looked embarrassed. If such gowns have to be worn, especially in an ambulatory setting, why can't they be better designed, and more protective of a patient's modesty? Doesn't anyone think of these things? Doesn't anyone care?

Having cancer involves many invasive tests and procedures, so it's important that doctors and others work hard to preserve a patient's sense of wholeness. Oddly, once the shock of having cancer wore off, I was grateful for any of these so-called invasions of my body—I saw them as positive steps—as long as my *dignity* was safeguarded.

August 1, 1996

It's hard to believe that I've had eleven radiation treatments so far, and am now past the halfway point. The daily trips to the hospital have been very easy because of the generous gift of a car service from both *Self* magazine and my neighbor, Carol (the friend I call "Earth Mother"). The hot, sticky days and the wet, chilly days all merged into comfortable days that did not disrupt my life very much at all. Accepting these gifts was hard for me (I just don't like to be beholden, I suppose), but once I did, I saw, of course, that to do so benefits not only the recipient, but the giver as well. "Earth Mother" told me it really helped her to be helping me (as she did during my chemo treatments, too).

I am not as tired as I expected to be, and the fatigue I do have seems to be just a continuation of the same side effect I had during chemo. Some days are better than others—some days I need to nap and/or go to bed very early—and some days I keep going until two A.M. It's very erratic. I try very hard to live life "normally," and lately it is only in my dreams that my anxieties seem to express themselves.

In one dream I was riding on a motorcycle (it's unclear whether I was the driver or passenger) and as I was going along, I noticed, in a fleeting glance, an unfamiliar man at the side of the road—and I rode on. Then I came to a stop sign and I saw this same man leaning against the sign. The motorcycle stopped, and then started down the road again, but the man grabbed me and pulled me off it. I awoke up with a start, disoriented and anxious. The evening before, my husband and I had had dinner with old friends whom I hadn't yet told about my cancer. Over the meal, after I did tell them, one of them bluntly asked me how long I had to live. "Five? seven? ten? years," I said haltingly. "But who really knows?" Clearly this conversation brought on the dream, I decided. My interpretation of it: I'm journeying along on my motorcycle (a motorcycle! taking a risk! I like that part). I'm aware of death (the man on the side of the road) being nearby—but I just go on with my living (as I'm doing). But then I come to a stop sign, and the man (death) grabs me off the road (of life) . Just like that. It's my time to "stop." In another dream, I was with my husband, Christopher, and my friend June, whom I call "Moon Beam" (I give some of my friends odd nicknames that stick, unfortunately for them) and we were going to a civic meeting in the neighborhood. I had trouble climbing the steps to a large government building, and I fell behind. Somehow I ended up alone on a dingy rooftop, and I couldn't find an exit (or entrance) into the building. Here the dream ended, and once again I awoke with a start. I lay awake in anguish—feeling a frightening sense of being left behind.

With great clarity I soon realized that this fear of being left behind is the real fear of dying. It's not the physical act of dying; no, it's not that at all; it's this other fear that is so dreadful: the fear of not only being left behind but being left out of the future. That is the pain, the misery, the sorrow. Later I admitted to myself and confided to Hugh that my greatest agony of all was thinking of Christopher with another woman. I cannot bear this. Yet I believe that until I can face it in some way I will not have come to terms with my dying. I think "Moon Beam" was in my dream not only because she is a community-minded friend and neighbor, but also because she met her present husband at her first husband's funeral, and married him just eight months later. I went to her wedding. I noticed her tears during the ceremony. "Do you know why I was crying?" she later asked me. "I'm not sure," I answered. "Well," she told me, "I was crying because I wanted Jonathan [her first husband] to be there with me and share my joy. It was a very strange sensation to be mourning and celebrating at the very same instant."

August 5, 1996

While on the Internet, I discovered an organization called the Lymphoma Research Foundation of America. I liked reading that most of their money goes toward financing research fellowships for doctors, and so I wrote for more details. I also found some information about a new type of radiation that uses a radioactive isotope of the metal yttrium to treat lymphoma patients who have relapsed after chemotherapy. I will ask Dr. Hayes about this the next time I see her. I decide to start a medical file called "The Future."

August 6, 1996

Dr. Hayes said that the yttrium-90 radiation, as it is called, is in phase-one trials, which is the earliest test on patients. It can be implanted in the body, she told me, and is not a conventional treatment. She emphasized that I've "barely seen the tip of the iceberg of available treatments. " Nonetheless, yttrium-90 will remain in "The Future," folder, for sure. As my cancer progresses over the years, I will have a folder full of options to discuss with my doctors.

August 7, 1996

I asked Denise, a radiation technician, if she ever gets depressed from doing her job. She hesitated, and then answered, "Sometimes."

August 8, 1996

Tomorrow is my last radiation treatment. But today I felt for the first time—really—that I can actually manage my cancer. Oh, I know I have talked about and thought about and have dealt with it, but the feeling today was different. I no longer dwell on my cancer's terminal aspects. My illness is now just part of the mix of everything about me, and I no longer twist with terror over its hold on me. I mean, Nancy, who is in the end-stage of her ovarian cancer, is still gaining weight. Life goes on. The body fights to save itself. "I'm going to go out with a bang," she said on the phone today. "I've got to go on living a life even though I have a tumor in my body that will never go away."

August 9, 1996

After my final radiation treatment today, I felt a sadness like the one that came over me after my last chemo session. I like when things are being done for my cancer. I feel safer. Now I'm set loose, so to speak, and have to wait three months for a PET scan to assess my fate. Still, I'm going to try to follow some of Dr. Wendy Harpham's advice: not to wait and see, but rather, "to live and see."

August 12, 1996

At my appointment with Dr. Mears today I asked him why there were no residents in his medical oncology department. He said there were, but in the clinic, not in the private practice. In the private practice, the care "is completely dictated by the attending," or senior doctor, although he conceded that "maybe there needs to be a total integration between the clinic and the private patients. It's a tough call." Then he added, "Somebody's got to be the first patient for a resident." I surprised myself by saying, "Not me." He laughed.

My regular blood test is now going to monitor something called my ESR rate, or erythrocyte sedimentation rate. "This is a rough gauge for lymphoma," Dr. Mears told me. "The test shows inflammation, and twenty is normal." He said that the test is helpful only if it is very high, say over fifty, although he also said, "It can be very high and not be lymphoma." In October of 1995, right before my diagnosis, my ESR rate was twelve. Today it's fifteen. "You're doing fine," Dr. Mears said.

I feel fine.

September 13, 1996

Today I had a follow-up appointment with my radiation oncologist, Dr. Mary Kay Hayes, who has now moved to New York Hospital. (Dr. Mears and I have decided that I will continue to see her—especially since Columbia-Presbyterian and New York Hospital have recently merged.)

When I mentioned that my back still hurt, Dr. Hayes told me something new and baffling: that my lower back tumor (my "malta") had been resting on bone. "But I never heard that before," I protested. "I always thought it was just sitting in the middle of some fatty tissue." She explained that there was a fuzzy area on an X-ray that showed lymphoma on the bone. "Radiation is causing some inflammation in the area," she went on, "but bone irritation is causing your pain." When I commented that it was a miracle that the cancer hadn't invaded my marrow, she nodded in agreement.

After I got home I called Dr. Mears, and he said that he would have a conversation with Dr. Hayes. He sounded very dubious about any bone involvement, and did not seem upset.

But I was.

October 2, 1996

Dr. Mears conceded today that my tumor was "so close that *maybe* it was into bone," but that he believes it was actually only "on top of bone," and then he added, diplomatically, "Dr. Hayes doesn't argue with us." (I liked the "us," meaning him and me.)

In other words, it's a close call. Because there's no marrow involvement, the bone isn't officially involved, I guess, even though the cancer did get very, very close to it.

I have a PET scan scheduled for November 4, and I'll have a great many answers after that test, and probably a great many questions, too.

October 3, 1996

Christopher and I decided not to celebrate our thirty-first anniversary, but we ended up having dinner with friends who found out at the end of the meal when the subject of marriage came up, and we owned up to our milestone.

One subject that did not come up was my cancer. I was overjoyed, because I am now going through a period of not wanting to talk about it. I have retreated, for reasons I do not yet fully understand, although I think they include my completing treatment, my coming up on a year since my diagnosis, and my acceptance of my new life.

October 5, 1996

Today I visited Diana, my elderly friend with lymphoma. Over the summer she became seriously ill, and now she is bedridden and knows she is dying. But we did not talk about that. It was not any form of denial that kept us from such a discussion—we have always discussed every subject that occurred to either of us—it was, instead, her unspoken but very present insistence that she go on living the moment. And so, at her request, I read aloud various items from the 100th anniversary issue of the *New York Times Book Review*. She especially liked the review of Freud's *A General Introduction to Psychoanalysis*. After a while, she closed her eyes, and eventually I asked her if I should leave. She nodded yes, and I kissed her on the forehead and went home, feeling a blankness all around me as I drove up Riverside Drive toward Riverdale.

October 10, 1996

Today I again visited Diana and, as I promised her I would, I read her parts of this journal. She wanted to hear more, but I had brought only a small section, thinking she would not be in the mood to listen for long because she is so weak. But I was wrong. (Never try to anticipate what the dying want, I have learned. My now ninety-one-year-old friend is not resisting death but still has some points of living to explore.) I told her I'd bring more of my journal in a few days. After a while she closed her eyes and when I asked if I should leave, this time she said no. She wanted me to sit beside her. I held her hand for over an hour, and felt an energy as strong as steel.

October 13, 1996

It seems that there are a lot of goodbyes this month. I visited my former sister-in-law, Nancy. "I'm dying," she told me in a peaceful voice. She no longer has a digestive system, but is in no pain because of medication she is using. "I'm looking forward to not waking up anymore," she said.

October 18, 1996

Today the new mattress that Christopher and I bought for our bed was delivered. At first I had said it was a waste of money to invest in an expensive item that I might not outlive, but when I saw the old mattress, torn and banged-up, being dragged out of the house, I knew the timing was right. I was not going to continue to sleep on lifeless springs.

October 23, 1996

At seven P.M. this evening Diana died from her lymphoma.

October 24, 1996

"Are you sure?" I said to Diana's son when he called to tell me that his mother had died. I never thought I would say such a stupid thing, but I did. I also found myself sympathizing with people who believe in spirits and go to séances to hear the voices of their departed relatives and friends. Already I miss Diana terribly—she was more than a friend: she was a sister and a mentor.

The cold air of this day was soundless.

October 30, 1996

I had a conversation today with the founder of the Lymphoma Research Foundation of America, Ellen Glesby Cohen. Ellen has had lymphoma for seven years ("the silent cancer," she calls it—"it just sits there") and she is an encyclopedia of lymphoma information. Her organization has contributed almost a million dollars to thirty-two lymphoma research projects in America.

I also recently learned about the Cure for Lymphoma Foundation, which also awards grants for cancer research at many places around the country. All of these groups, including the Leukemia Society of America, are doing critical, effective funding and educational work; it is both gratifying and reassuring to know that such organizations exist and are looking for a cancer cure. It is only now that I can focus on such organizations and think about ways I might help them.

November 4, 1996

I had my PET scan today. A neighbor had asked if she could go with me, but I said I wanted to go alone. Later

I called her back to be sure I hadn't hurt her feelings. But I really did want to be in the hospital by myself.

The test took a little over four hours this time. I'll know where I stand in twenty-four (or so) hours.

November 7, 1996

Dr. Mears, who got my PET report only today, said that my scans are "clear." There is "some" inflammation in my lower back, but "this is thought to be the after-effects of radiation."

"Am I in remission?" I asked Dr. Mears.

"Yes," he replied happily, adding, "I knew you would be."

November 11, 1996

Christopher came with me to my appointment with Dr. Mears today. Dr. Mears explained to us that it "could be several years before my lymphoma recurs," but he also said that there is "one chance in fifty that the remission could last forever."

I talked to him about his children and he said that his daughter is taking driving lessons, and that his son is in the school band. I love the expression on Dr. Mears's face when he is discussing his family.

Dr. Mears asked us what we were reading. I showed him the book I brought along, *Architect of Desire*, by Susanna Lassard. "It's a haunting, unusual memoir," I told him, and explained that the author "was" the great-granddaughter of Stanford White. "She still is," Christopher corrected me. "Does he always do that?" Dr. Mears asked. "Yes," my husband and I answered in unison. "Well, I'd want to smash him if he did that to me," Dr. Mears said good-naturedly (I think). "My wife often does," Christopher answered, his blue-green eyes sparkling. We all laughed.

We all laughed.

I loved that Dr. Mears was comfortable enough with us—and my future—to tease us. When we parted, he looked at me and said, "I'll see you in three months." I marked it down in my pocket calendar. "You know," he said, as we walked toward the exit, "you can live with this lymphoma quite successfully and not be too frightened that it will kill you."

AFTERWORD

The title of this journal began with a misunderstanding, or rather, my misreading of a quote from *Romeo and Juliet*: "How oft when men are at the point of death they have been merry, which their keepers call a lightening before death." I first read "lightening" as "lightning," which my Random House dictionary defines as the "luminous, electric discharge in the atmosphere . . . produced in thunderstorms," and not the word that Shakespeare no doubt meant, which means "to lessen the load of or upon, to make less burdensome, to cheer or gladden." Still, the dictionary also says under the definition of "lighten," "it thundered and lightened for hours," and under the definition for "lightning," it states that the word can be a variation of "lightening." Confusing? I guess so. But, in fact all the meanings have relevance when it comes to living with cancer. There is the danger, naturally, and there is the relief that I have written about. So my initial misreading made a kind of sense, and gives the quote even

greater significance now that I am facing my first recur-
rence. In early June of 1998, a two-and-a-half inch tumor
was discovered in my left pleural/thoracic region, and I
will begin treatment soon.

But for almost two years, I often forgot about my cancer. When I expressed concern over this to a friend who
happens to be a doctor, she said, "Fine. As long as you
don't forget your checkups!" Perhaps this ought to be the
goal of anyone with a chronic disease or disorder: remember, but not all the time. I'm trying to follow my own advice now that I'm out of remission.

Actually, I rarely tell new people I meet about my cancer, and I find myself reluctant even to mention this book.
I talk about other projects I am working on (I've aban-
doned the "Fundamental Women" idea for two others),
but often I leave my journal out. This may seem like my
denying that cancer is a part of who I am now, yet it really isn't. By putting cancer behind me (or beside me) I
am reaffirming my goal as a writer to keep moving ahead.
This is the hardest task of all for anyone with cancer, yet
the one that matters most. It affirms the future without
denying the past. Still, moving ahead when you have cancer is like running through lightning. There are all kinds
of scenes in your memory and in the distance, but all you
can see is an intense flashing, and all you can hear is a
blasting crack of thunder, as the storm makes its way over
you, over you, until it passes, until the next time, or until it's over.

Many of the people I mention in this journal are still

alive. The woman with the maroon tee shirt and matching leggings, the neatly coiffed ash-blond woman, and the bronze-skinned woman with fuchsia lipstick who often wore a floppy black felt hat with a large pink rose on it. New drugs and therapies are keeping people in remission longer and longer. (Since my own original diagnosis, Rituxan, a new drug specifically for indolent non-Hodgkin's lymphomas, has come on the market, and I will be using it, along with fludarabine, the chemotherapy I used before. The cancer world is changing and getting closer to cures each second.) Faith, my friend with deadly mesothelioma, is doing well because of new chemotherapies. So is the editor and writer Michael Korda, a prostate cancer survivor, and the actress Barbara Barrie, a colon cancer survivor, who told me on New Year's Day, 1996: "Your cancer will bring you gifts." And it has. Dr. Wendy Schlessel Harpham, an eight-year lymphoma survivor, offered to send me a copy of her first book, *Diagnosis: Cancer*, when she read that I had trouble finding it. This act of generosity began an important new friendship, a close relationship I treasure. We now communicate almost daily by e-mail or telephone, chatting about our families, our writing, our worries, our ideas, books we have read or want to read—or want to write—and yes, our cancer. I have found that for me, this kind of one-on-one support system works best. I'm just not a joiner, although I've listed in "Suggestions for Further Reading and Thinking" some places to find the excellent support groups that are around. There is no one right way to do anything when it comes to cancer—as long as your doctor knows what you are doing.

I have said that perhaps when the urge to write everything down went away (although I doubted it ever would) it might mean that I had adjusted to my new life. Well, during my remission, I didn't keep a journal on any regular basis, although I wrote extensive notes about all of my tests and doctors' visits, checked the Internet weekly for cancer news, and kept adding newspaper and magazine articles to my now bulging medical file labeled "The Future." And I started a series of letters I call "A Thousand Letters to the Future," messages I am leaving for my family to read after I die. This is my way of not being left out of the future, I suppose. But lately I have begun keeping a journal again. Have I "unadjusted" to life with cancer? I don't think so. Wendy Harpham suspects that my losing the urge to write about my cancer might have been a reflection of my being in remission. I agree, and believe that my new urge to write everything down simply reflects my need as a writer "to cover" the new and unsettling events that are happening around me.

Cancer has also brought me another gift, one that is harder to describe. It came from the Hasidic family I mentioned, whose piousness inspired me when I was undergoing my first round of chemotherapy. After the wife died of leukemia, someone—I think it even might have been Dr. Mears—showed the young widower my journal entries about his wife, and he called me. He told me that what I had written had enabled him to cry for the first time. He asked permission to include my words in a memorial book he was assembling for private printing. He also said that as a result of his wife's death, he was determined to go to medical school. He also wanted to meet me, and introduce me to his son—his son! On a warm, summer day in June of 1997, I met this compassionate and serious-minded young rabbinical student and his fourteen-month-old baby. His mother-in-law came, too, and I learned that she was her only grandson's primary caretaker while her son-in-law continued to study the Torah. Sitting on my backyard terrace, I saw with pleasure that this miraculous baby was in good hands: a loving grandmother and a good father, who even changed diapers! He gave me a copy of the memorial book that had been recently printed. Later, when I read it, I saw what an exceptional young woman his wife had been. At the same time I wondered why I was still so involved with the lives of these people I barely knew. And why did I feel so honored when the young widower called me a year later to tell me that he had some good news? He was getting married to someone he had met through mutual friends, and I would be invited to the festivities. After the wedding in Israel, the baby would be coming to live with them, "so he can have a fresh start," he said. His fiancée, a twenty-two-year-old woman from Brussels, would be a fine mother to his son. Yet I found myself worrying about his first wife's mother having to give up her grandson. Would she be able to visit him as often as she wished? Then I remembered that when I asked the young husband earlier about remarriage he had said that when that time came, his son would be lucky because he would have six grandparents instead of four. Still, I thought about calling his former mother-in-law on the day of the wedding, but to express what? Sadness over a joyful wedding? Or to say that life must go on, which she surely already understands?

My husband thinks that my being taken seriously by an Orthodox Jew feels like a special gift because of my ambivalent feelings about my non-practicing Judaism. He might be right. In many ways, I envy the ability of this family to observe their religion so passionately and strictly. But I'm afraid it's not for me. Still, I wish I could attend the wedding in Israel, a country I have never visited. And I look forward to receiving the promised photographs of the bride and groom. And I hope to hear word that the baby boy is flourishing, has brothers and sisters, and that the young husband has become a doctor. I want to remain part of this family because I feel part of it.

This, too, is what cancer does for you: it gives you communities you didn't have before, or ever thought you wanted to be part of, privileges you never thought you'd use, and friendships that are worth going into the lightning for. It can make wives love husbands more, husbands love wives more, children love their parents more, and parents love their children more. It intensifies, energizes, and electrifies all of life, all around us, all the time.   —June 20, 1998

SUGGESTIONS FOR FURTHER READING AND THINKING

BOOKS ABOUT CANCER THAT I KEEP ON THE SHELF OVER MY BED

Babcock, Elise NeeDell, *When Life Becomes Precious: A Guide for Loved Ones and Friends of Cancer Patients*. New York: Bantam Books, 1997
§   Good, practical blueprints for coping.

Barrie, Barbara, *Don't Die of Embarrassment*. (Formerly *Second Act*, published in 1997). New York: Scribner's: 1999.
§   Essential reading for colon cancer survivors. Barrie is now a spokesperson for Convatec, the ostomy equipment manufactured by Bristol Myers Squibb.

Benjamin, Harold H. *The Wellness Community/Guide to Fighting for*

Recovery from Cancer. Rev. ed. New York: G. P. Putnam, 1995.
§ Useful strategies for cancer patients.

Harpham, Wendy Schlessel, M.D. *Diagnosis: Cancer: Your Guide Through the First Few Months.* Rev. ed. New York: W. W. Norton, 1998.
———. *After Cancer: A Guide to Your New Life.* New York: Harper Perennial, 1995.
———. *When a Parent Has Cancer: A Guide to Caring for Your Children.* New York: HarperCollins, 1997.
§ No one writes better about cancer than Dr. Harpham. These books are absolutely essential for every cancer patient's library. Her bibliography and resource sections are also excellent.

Hoffman, Barbara J.D., and Fitzhugh Mullan, M.D. *Charting the Journey: A Cancer Survivor's Almanac.* New York: Chronimed Publishing, 1996.
§ Very useful and informative guide, especially regarding insurance and work issues.

Korda, Michael. *Man-to-Man: Surviving Prostate Cancer.* New York: Random House, 1996; Vintage Books, 1997.
§ A powerful account by a survivor.

Lang, Susan S., and Richard B. Patt, M.D. *You Don't Have to Suffer: A Complete Guide to Relieving Cancer Pain for Patients and Their Families.* New York: Oxford University Press, 1994.
§ Very sensible and clear.

Morra, Marion, and Eve Potts. *Choices.* New York: Avon Books, 1994.
§ A first-rate source book.

Murphy, Gerald P., M.D., Lois B. Morris, and Dianne Lange. *The American Cancer Society's Informed Decisions:The Complete Book*

of Cancer Diagnosis, Treatment and Recovery. New York: Viking, 1997.
§   Comprehensive and state-of-the art.

Steingraber, Sandra. *Living Downstream: An Ecologist Looks at Cancer and the Environment.* New York: Addison Wesley Longman, 1997.
§   A poet's investigation.

Weinberg, Robert A. *Racing to the Beginning of the Road: The Search for the Origin of Cancer.* New York: Crown Publishing Group,1996.
§   The inside story of cancer research by the head of MIT's famed Whitehead Institute.

Zakarian, Beverly. *The Activist Cancer Patient: How to Take Charge of Your Treatment.* New York: Wiley, 1996.
§   Great advice.

GOOD PLACES TO CONTACT FOR INFORMATION AND SUPPORT GROUPS

National Cancer Institute
9000 Rockville Pike
Bethesda, Md. 20892
800–4–CANCER
www.nci.nih.gov

American Cancer Society
1599 Clifton Road, N.E.
Atlanta, Ga. 30329
404–320–3333
800–227–2345
www.cancer.org

Cure for Lymphoma Foundation
215 Lexington Avenue
New York, N.Y. 10016
212–213–9595
email: infocfl@aol.com
www.cfl.org

Leukemia Society of America (Leukemia, lymphoma, myeloma)
600 Third Avenue
New York, N.Y. 10016
212–573–8484
800–955–4LSA
www.leukemia.org

Lymphoma Research Foundation of America
8800 Venice Blvd. #207
Los Angeles, Calif. 90034
310–204–7040
email: LRFA@aol.com
www.lymphoma.org

National Coalition for Cancer Survivorship
1010 Wayne Avenue
Silver Springs, Md. 20910
301–650–8868
www.cansearch.org

(OTHER) CYBERSITES I VISIT OFTEN

American Medical Association
www.ama-assn.org

"CancerNet," National Cancer Institute
www.cancernet.nci.nih. gov

"CanSearch," National Coalition for Cancer Survivorship
www.CanSearch.org

The Lancet, a British medical journal
www.thelancet.com

www.medmatrix.org/spages/oncology. asp

"Mayo Health Oasis," The Mayo Clinic
www.mayo.edu

Massachusetts General Hospital Cancer Center
"MedWeb:Oncology"
www.cancer.mgh.harvard.edu

The New England Journal of Medicine
www.nejm.org/content/index asp

"OncoLink"
www.oncolink.upenn.edu